The Bisected Brain

Neuroscience Series

EDITOR:
Arnold Towe, University of Washington

PREVIOUS TITLE:

Physiological Basis of the Alpha Rhythm
by Per Andersen (University of Oslo) and
Sven Andersson (University of Gothenburg)

The Bisected Brain

MICHAEL S. GAZZANIGA
*Department of Psychology,
New York University
Washington Square, New York*

APPLETON-CENTURY-CROFTS
EDUCATIONAL DIVISION   MEREDITH CORPORATION
NEW YORK

Copyright © 1970 by MEREDITH CORPORATION

All rights reserved. This book, or parts thereof, must not be used or reproduced in any manner without written permission. For information address the publisher, Appleton-Century-Crofts, Educational Division, Meredith Corporation, 440 Park Avenue South, New York, New York, 10016.

713-2

Library of Congress Catalog Card Number: 77-105426

PRINTED IN THE UNITED STATES OF AMERICA
390-35278-0

For my father,
DANTE ACHILLES GAZZANIGA, M.D.

Preface

The mysteries of the mind remain as elusive today as ever before. While there have been great technologic advances in the study of the brain, yielding enormous amounts of data on its physical and psychologic characteristics, the old problem of relating mind to brain in a reasonable fashion remains unaccomplished. It is not that the researcher lacks the will or even the know-how. Rather, it is clearly a problem of not knowing what are the proper and most important questions to ask. We have but scratched the surface and are still looking for a way to crack the brain code in an orderly fashion.

The field of brain research is so enormous, so complicated, and so prolific that it is almost impossible to introduce any subject in a scholarly fashion by pointing to the antecedent studies which clearly spell out the nature of the next logical question for inquiry. One quickly gains the impression that for every issue there are two opposite views with authoritative investigators on each side. Moreover, as in almost no other field of scientific investigation, what looks good today will look weak tomorrow. Indeed, because of this more than one scientist has confessed a certain feeling of futility in reporting his research.

These problems, combined with the overall information explosion of recent years, have splintered the brain code investigators so much that rare is the study that talks to all involved in the effort. It is still less frequent when one man is responsible for contributing unique and pioneering studies two or three times. Roger W. Sperry has, of course, and with a genius and excellence that will not soon be matched. Moving from his breathtaking experiments on neurospecificity into the discovery of the split-brain (along with his graduate student R. E. Myers) is a contribution of incredible magnitude. There can be no serious discussion of the neurologic basis of learning and memory until one has grasped the implication of Sperry's early work on the nature of the developing nervous system. Paradoxically, the split-brain preparation is a discovery of another kind. Phenomenologically it is devastating, but its hard implications for a theory of brain function, if there are any, are not yet apparent. Yet, the enormity of the research tool is clearly leading to the view that anything you can do I can do better with a split.

This book is about split-brains. It will review critically much of the recent work (though not all of it) on the subjects which are of special interest to me. I will forego a historical survey of the ideas and events that lead up to its discovery for a brief history has been printed elsewhere (Sperry 1961).

There are many people who helped in this effort. The studies on the human cases would not have been possible without the generous cooperation of Doctors P. J. Vogel and J. E. Bogen of the California College of Medicine. At Caltech, of course, one could always count on the guidance, counsel, experience, support, and judgment of Professor Sperry in all phases of research. C. R. Hamilton, R. F. Mark, C. B. Trevarthen, and many others contributed invaluable suggestions. At the University of California, Santa Barbara, I was generously supported by the United States Public Health Service as well as the University of California. Many helpful suggestions and criticisms on the manuscript were made by Lila Ghent Braine. Also David Premack and Arthur Schwartz offered many insights into problems in behavior and language function. Finally, I would like to acknowledge the tireless assistance of my secretary Melanie McLees.

Contents

PREFACE / *vii*

1. Introduction: What is a Split-Brain? / *1*
2. Methods and Procedures of Split-Brain Research / *5*
3. Sensory-Sensory Integration / *19*
4. Sensory-Motor Control Mechanisms / *33*
5. Callosal Code / *59*
6. Psychologic and Neurologic Effects of Cerebral Bisection in Man / *74*
7. Cerebral Dominance and Lateral Specialization / *128*
8. Early Versus Late Lesions—More Apparent Than Real / *135*
9. An Overview and New Directions / *141*

REFERENCES / *160*

INDEX / *169*

Illustrations

Figure 1. Mid-sagittal view of human brain / *3*
Figure 2. The animal neurosurgical chair / *6*
Figure 3. Animal neurosurgical instruments / *8*
Figure 4. Scale and placement of neurosurgical instruments with relation to the actual brain structures / *10*
Figure 5. Cross-section of a monkey brain / *12*
Figure 6. Cat-training box / *14*
Figure 7. Behavioral training apparatus / *16*
Figure 8. Sketch of automated testing apparatus / *17*
Figure 9. Automated visual-tactile testing device / *23*
Figure 10. Visual-tactile association performed by a split-brain patient / *26*
Figure 11. Strategies employed by the left hand for detecting features of objects / *28*
Figure 12. Motor responses to verbal commands in Case I / *38*
Figure 13. Motor responses to verbal commands in Case II / *40*
Figure 14. Hand positions flashed to left or right hemisphere to test control ability of each half-brain / *42*
Figure 15. Deep-split surgery in the midline, down into the medulla / *45*
Figure 16. Brain of a monkey showing cortical lesion / *46*
Figure 17. Automated testing device for measuring accuracy of reaching / *49*
Figure 18. Representative data of control monkeys / *53*
Figure 19. Data on split-brain monkeys / *55*
Figure 20. Test apparatus for eye movements / *57*

Figure 21. Eye movement recordings of normal and split-brain patients / 58
Figure 22. Sagittal sections of monkey brains / 64
Figure 23. Callosal units with simple and complex visual receptive fields / 69
Figure 24. Relations of receptive fields of callosal units to the vertical meridian of the visual field / 70
Figure 25. Retention of motor coordination after split-brain surgery / 79
Figure 26. Points of stimulation on palmar surface of hand / 83
Figure 27. Test of position sense / 86
Figure 28. Test of intermanual tactile discrimination / 86
Figure 29. Test of visual function / 91
Figure 30. Apparatus to measure reaction time to visual discrimination / 97
Figure 31. Examples of written responses after split-brain surgery / 99
Figure 32. Attempts to arrange blocks on a table / 100
Figure 33. Nature of subject's response to visual stimuli / 106
Figure 34. Apparatus producing stimuli with emotional quality / 108
Figure 35. Course of pupil dilation / 111
Figure 36. Tests of ability to handle visual information / 112
Figure 37. Schematic view of Dodge Tachistoscope / 113
Figure 38. Extent of lesion necessary to produce state of functional blindness in split-brain monkey / 149
Figure 39. Test of visually guided behavior in splenium-intact, chiasm-sectioned monkey / 150
Figure 40. Pathway for intrahemispheric transmission of visual information / 152

The Bisected Brain

1

Introduction: What is a Split-Brain?

Situated dead center in the middle of the brain is the largest and most mysterious information transmission system in the world—the corpus callosum. With it intact, the two halves of the body have no secrets from one another. With it sectioned, the two halves become two different conscious mental spheres, each with its own experienced base and control system for behavioral operations. Just as conjoined twins are two different people sharing a common body, the callosum-sectioned human has two separate conscious spheres sharing a common brain stem, head, and body. Unbelievable as this may seem, this is the flavor of a long series of experimental studies first carried out in the cat and monkey. More recently observations of this kind have been possible in human patients.

Consider what has been said. The natural organization of the mammalian brain is such that a slice of the surgeon's knife through the midline commissures produces two separate, but equal, cognitive systems each with its own abilities to learn, emote, think, and act. The now classic experiment worked out by Myers and Sperry (1953) demonstrated that midline sectioning of the optic chiasm and the corpus callosum and anterior commissure in the cat produced an animal who was unable, using the untrained eye, to perform a visual discrimination learned through the opposite eye. Thus, when a cat with a patch over one eye is trained and overtrained on a pattern discrimination, testing of the untrained eye finds the animal unable to perform the task. In point of fact, the second half-brain must learn the discrimination from the beginning. Comparison of the learning curves between the two hemispheres shows them to be nearly identical. This finding, which gave rise to the double-brain phenomenon, startled the neuropsychology community. Here for the first time in the history of experimental psychology, surgical disconnection of a brain structure had resulted in a complete breakdown of communication of high-order "mental" properties between brain areas. Yet, the surgery itself in no way produced easily detectable abnormalities with respect to the everyday behavior of the organism!

To take a specific example, let us examine the behavior of a split-brain monkey during a visual discrimination transfer task. Prior to the test, the animal has undergone midline section of the corpus callosum, anterior and hippocampal commissures, and optic chiasm. Postoperatively, when the animal's vision is restricted to the right eye, only the right hemisphere receives visual information, and when visual information is restricted to the left eye, the converse is true. Typically, the animal views the visual situation through one eye, and either or both hands are free to make the response. After training and considerable overtraining on the visual-pattern discrimination, the trained eye is occluded and the untrained eye is tested. What one sees on the first transfer trials is a complete naiveté with respect to the test stimulus. The animal's response latencies and his examination of the stimulus panels is reminiscent of the kind of behavior seen when the first eye was learning the discrimination. In short, the animal shows no knowledge of the problem through the untrained eye, and proceeds to learn the discrimination at the normal rate.

Of course, if such tests were run on chiasm-sectioned, callosum-intact monkeys, nearly complete transfer would be observed. Here, when a monkey is trained on a discrimination through one eye, the untrained eye can usually perform the task with little or no deficit apparent.

WHAT IS A SPLIT-BRAIN?

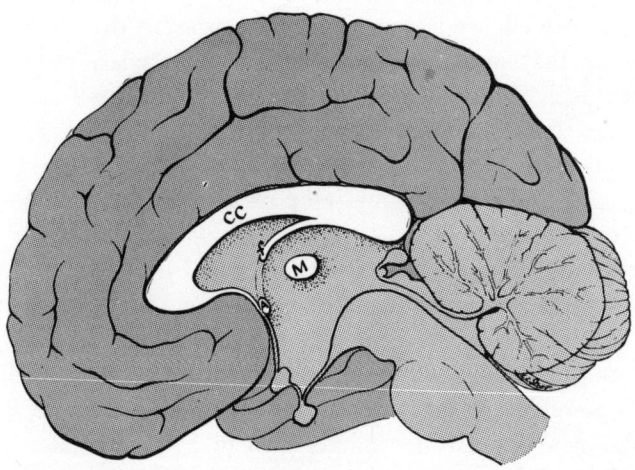

Figure 1. Mid-sagittal view of human brain. The major interhemispheric communication systems are the corpus callosum (CC) and anterior commissure (A). Both of these structures are sectioned in patients operated on for surgical control of epileptic seizures. M, massa intermedia; f, fornix.

This same kind of very simple transfer test has been repeatedly run on human patients with bisected brains (Fig. 1). In tactile tests, for example, the patients would be presented with objects out of view of the left hand. In a preliminary trial they would be asked to describe the objects, but they could not. This is because the stereognostic information for the left hand is projected to the right hemisphere (Chapter 6); and it, of course, remains isolated there because of the deconnection surgery, thus leaving the left speech hemisphere ignorant of the nature of the stimulus. On subsequent trials, the patients were taught to retrieve but one of the objects. Each time they would pick up the positive stimulus, a bell would ring. After perfect responding was established and stabilized over 30 trials, the patient would again be allowed to make a verbal guess. Here again it was a question of the left hemisphere trying to figure out what was going on in the right, with the result that only chance performance was obtained. Also, in the transfer test the right hand proved unable to respond to the object correctly. In a simple sense then, the right hand did not know what was going on in the left hand, under these lateralized testing conditions.

It is the cerebral commissures, then, which are responsible for interhemispheric transfer of learning and memory. Put differently, with the callosum and anterior commissure intact, there is perceptual unity;

with the commissures sectioned, each half-brain behaves independently. Moreover, as we will see later on, it is the posterior fifth of the callosum together with the anterior commissure which is solely responsible for the interhemispheric transfer of visual learning. These specific brain structures are among the few examples in neuropsychology where one can say with certainty that a better understanding of the neural and coding logic of this system would take us a long way in understanding the brain code in general.

Remarkable as it seemed to Myers and Sperry when they made their first observation on this kind of task some 15 years ago, the split-brain phenomenon remains as one of neuropsychology's truly exciting and most enigmatic discoveries. In addition to the phenomenon being used as a powerful research tool, the basic findings raise intriguing philosophic questions. Do two minds exist in one head following surgical manipulation? Are the mental properties of the normal human held in duplicate so that disconnection of the cerebral hemispheres results in two conscious mental spheres each with its own set of output controls? If the foregoing is true, does this present difficulties for traditional views relating mind to brain?

In the following chapters, there will be an effort to consider some of the major problems in neuropsychology using the split-brain approach. Out of these discussions and considerations, hopefully, will come answers to some of the questions posed in the foregoing, as well as others raised along the way.

2

Methods and Procedures of Split-Brain Research

Many of the surgical as well as behavioral training techniques used in split-brain research are unique and of a special kind. In this chapter several of these procedures will be described. Those not concerned with the "how-to-do-it" aspects of the subject ought to pass on to the remaining chapters, which deal with specific problems in neuropsychology.

The surgical procedures and equipment used to perform split-brain surgery were first developed by Myers for the cat (Myers, 1955). Many modifications have been made since this pioneering work. For the most part, techniques described in the following are more or less similar to those currently used by most investigators in the area and were developed largely by Sperry (1968a).

Animal Neurosurgical Chair

The basic design of the animal surgical chair allows for maximum flexibility in positioning the head. As can be seen from Figure 2, a

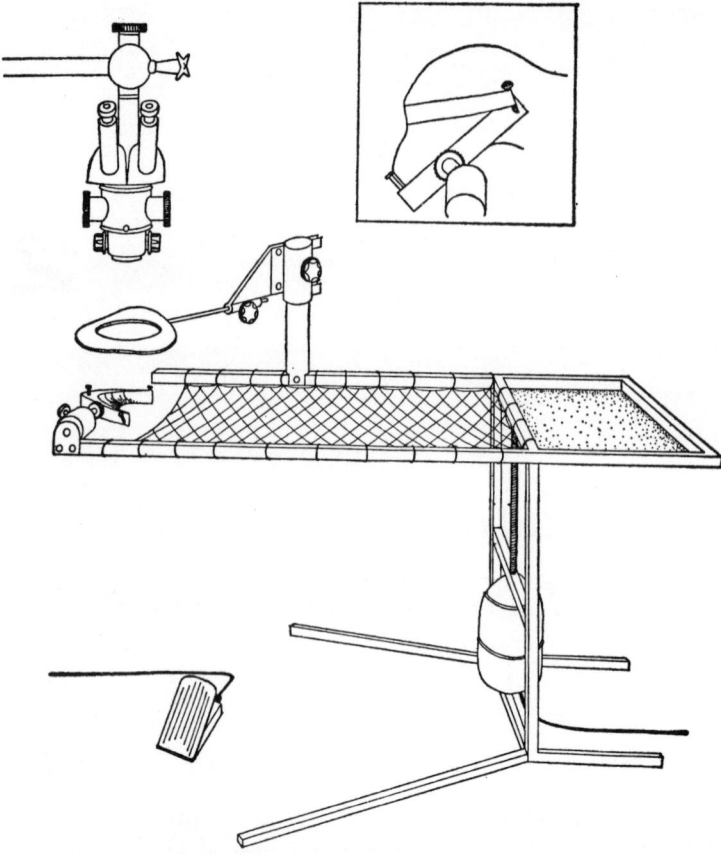

Figure 2. The hammock-shaped neurosurgical chair allows maximum flexibility in the positioning of the head. The head, as shown in the insert, is mounted on a form-fit plexiglass ladle and taped along the lateral and posterior surfaces of the skull. The ball-and-socket joint enables adjustment of head position. The entire unit is mounted on the side arm of the L-shaped chair as seen in the large sketch. Vertical adjustment of the chair is easily managed with the reversible motor, controlled by a foot switch shown at the bottom. An adjustable knob on the irregularly shaped head holder is used for positioning of the hands at the best possible level.

universal ball-and-socket joint makes necessary only one adjusting knob for the positioning of the head at almost any angle relative to the surgeon. For routine commissurotomy, the head holder is held parallel to the vertical bars. For deep-split surgery, it is turned down at a right angle, allowing for a clear approach to the base of the skull and the fourth ventricle.

On the horizontal bar opposite the surgeon an adjustable, flat, wide, oval hand rest is attached. This allows for steady and even control of the hands when holding instruments in positions deep in the brain. It too is adjustable to allow for any inclination relative to the head.

The body of the animal rests on a fishnet type hammock, which is suspended between the horizontal bars. It may be raised or lowered to assure the most advantageous position for the animal's respiration.

This unit allows the surgeon to sit down during the entire operation. The head is rigidly taped to a plexiglass head holder, and the animal is, of course, completely draped and the scalp shaved in routine fashion for sterile surgery. EKG, body temperature, and respiration are sometimes monitored, but usually are not.

The entire chair is welded to a screw drive geared into a reversible motor attached to a foot control, which allows for both upward and downward movement. This feature is most useful for adjusting the distance of the animal from the microscope. Previously, the dissecting microscope itself was equipped with a similar reversible drive system, but this proved to be less efficient than the present method. Now the surgeon need not move his head up or down with the microscope but rather keeps his gaze constant and moves the animal in the chair up or down along the focal plane.

Surgical Instruments

It is imperative for split-brain surgery that a dissecting microscope be used. It is equally important that the surgeon use the surgical tools made for the job. By and large, these instruments have been designed and developed by Sperry (1968a). The fine points of design are constantly being changed and modified. The more important pieces are shown in Figure 3.

The hemisphere dividers are made out of 0.031-inch[1] spring stainless steel. They are bent in such a fashion as to have the tips rest with a half-inch separation. When squeezed together they fall perfectly in line and can be easily lowered into the brain. Upon carefully relaxing the grip, the tips move back 1/8 to 1/4 inch retracting the tissue around them, thereby clearing away an adequate surgical field.

The suckers are made out of standard hypodermic needles, which, as a rule, are bent at a 45° angle. The tip is usually ground down and

[1] 1 inch = 2.54 cm (approximately).

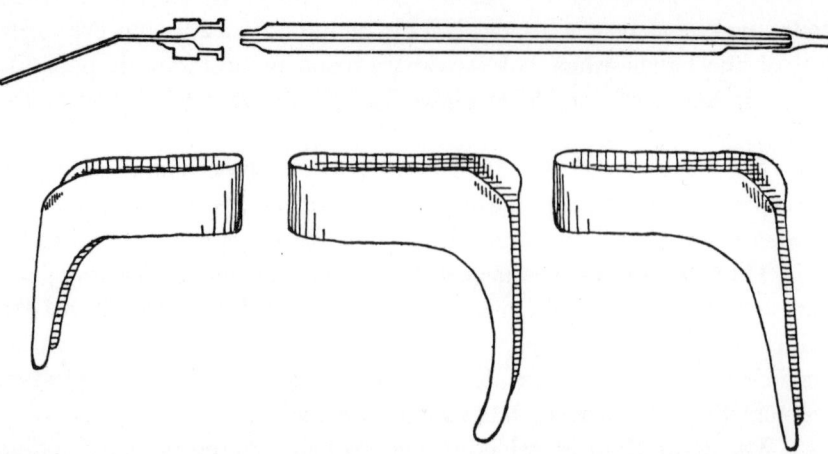

Figure 3. Most of these animal neurosurgical instruments were designed by Sperry. The three specula below allow for easy hemisphere separation in the monkey. A smaller variety is used in the cat. Above is a typical sucker used in aspirating and cutting the commissural systems.

made dull. Sometimes, however, the tip is sharpened so that it may serve both as a sucker and as a knife. The suckers themselves fit into a stainless steel handle, which is connected to a vacuum pump. There are many different shapes and sizes of suckers.

For cutting the chiasm as well as other deep structures, special knives have been developed. These are bent at a variety of angles depending on the job to be carried out. By and large, they are modified to order and made from basic instruments.

Operation—General Procedure

There are many different overall approaches in split-brain surgery. Each surgeon develops his own individual methods and procedures for the operation. By and large, it is self-taught and at first the surgical procedure seems difficult. While cutting the callosum is routine and rather simple, especially in the monkey, complications arise when surgery includes the anterior commissure and optic chiasm. Clear as the relations seem to be in the anatomy book, the live brain plays many tricks on the surgeon first attempting this operation. With a little persistence and patience, however, the relationships and midline topography form a clear picture, with the result that the entire split-brain operation becomes a rather routine and simple procedure. The following is a step-by-step description of the operation in the monkey.

After the animal has been anesthetized, the head shaved, cleansed, and mounted in the head holder on the chair, the operative field is draped. A three-inch midline incision is then made starting from the orbital ridge, the skin is retracted back and clamped to a towel, and the periosteum is scraped back to the temporal muscles on each side.

A medium-sized, rectangular bone segment is then removed; it is generally 1½ inches long and 1 inch wide, with ¼ inch falling over the midline. Anteriorally, the edge starts about ⅜ to ½ inch in front of the apex of the coronal suture and extends back for the 1½ inches. While there are a variety of procedures of freeing the bone, one of the simplest procedures is to drill a series of ¹⁄₁₆-inch holes with a dental drill around the circumference of the rectangle. Subsequently, these holes are connected together with bone cutters and the bone segment snapped out. The bone segment is then wrapped in gauze which has been soaked in saline, and is set aside for later replacement.

In retracting the dura mater, a slit is made slightly above the lower extent of the cranial opening and extended along the entire length. A flap is prepared by cutting along the anterior and posterior borders of the opening, and is then turned back to the midline. Care is taken to avoid extending the dural section into the sagittal sinus. Occasionally, there are adhesions between the dura mater and communicating veins going into the sinus. Rather than trying to tease the dura away from the veins and risk rupture, a slit is made in the dura on each side of the vein and it is then turned back in multiple sections. Cottonoid pieces, soaked in saline, are placed over the exposed dura and over the exposed cortex.

The number of communicating veins into the sagittal sinus from the cortex varies from animal to animal, but there are rarely more than one or two. In general, the surgeon can easily work around them and leave them intact. Ligation of large veins often results in severe swelling of the exposed hemisphere. Occasionally, however, when ligation has been necessary, little or no swelling has resulted.

The speculum and a small gauge sucker are then lowered down between the hemispheres (Fig. 4). In the monkey, there are rarely adhesions between the medial wall of the retracted hemisphere and the falx in the posterior callosal region. Quite frequently, there is a large arterial plexus over both the splenium and the body of the callosum just dorsal to the anterior tip of the massa intermedia. Here

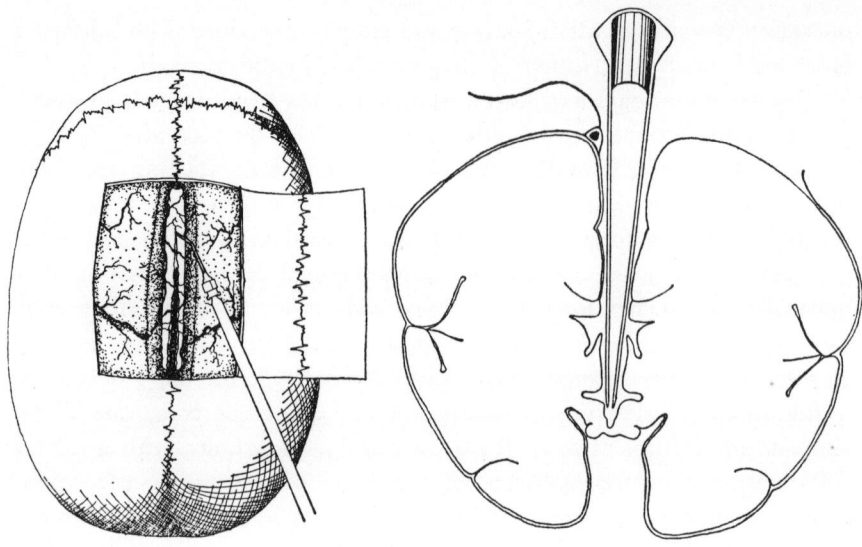

Figure 4. Scale and placement of neurosurgical instruments with relation to the actual brain structures are indicated. The sketch at the right shows the extent of the intrusion of the speculum. The other sketch depicts the cranial opening and shows the small sucker in place between the hemispheres for both aspiration and suction of callosal tissue.

again, care is taken not to rupture these arteries, and with the aid of the dissecting microscope and special surgical tools it is easily possible to avoid ruptures.

Sectioning the callosum is accomplished by making slight brush-like movements with the small gauge sucker into the callosal tissue, each penetration extending down but a fraction of the total depth. In general, the subcallosal midline structures and landmarks necessary for successful surgery are most clearly evident when sectioning proceeds in a caudal-rostral direction. When the callosum has been completely penetrated in the splenial area, cerebrospinal fluid seeps upward and momentarily clouds the field. This is easily sucked away and one immediately sees the choroid plexus of the third ventricle. As sectioning proceeds anteriorally, the massa intermedia is clearly visualized beneath a thin membrane ventral to the choroid plexus. The gray color of the massa intermedia is strikingly apparent in relation to the callosum and other surrounding brain structures. As mentioned above, there is usually a heavy plexus of communicating arteries at the anterior tip of the massa intermedia. This is a critical landmark in the surgical procedure. At this point, the surgeon should be confident that the midline is obtained and that he has moved sufficiently anteriorally to be at the rostral curvature of the massa intermedia. With the animal's head positioned level and perpendicular to the table and the surgical microscope set in a vertical position, lowering of the speculum and the sucker through the light membrane at this point clearly reveals the interventricular foramen and more ventrally the anterior commissure. Again, care should be made to visualize the anterior commissure in the midline. (It is easy to become confused at this point and probe into the third ventricle. The anterior commissure can be sectioned in this way, but for a clear view of the chiasm the surgeon must then make his way back into the midline by a medial move. This usually results in some damage in the hypothalamic and preoptic area.)

When the midline is observed and the anterior commissure is visualized and sectioned from the midline position, then a straight downward movement of the speculum at the level of the anterior commissure will clearly and easily reveal the optic chiasm, which lies just a millimeter or two posterior to the anterior commissure. After clearing the field of any fluid, the chiasm is clearly visualized and sectioned down the midline with the aid of one of the specially designed surgical knives. The knife is lowered into the tissue and then run anteriorally and superiorally along the sphenoid bone. The section is then checked by lowering the speculum into the chiasm, and with the small gauge sucker completeness of section can be verified. Subsequently, the instruments are withdrawn and the major remaining task is to complete the sectioning of the anterior portions of the callosum.

At this point there is some variability in the success of splitting the callosum and septum in the midline. Frequently, the callosum is sectioned and the septum is left intact; skilled surgeons can perform either task with relative ease.

When the operation is complete, the retracted hemisphere is gently pushed toward the midline. All bleeders are stopped and the dura is laid back over the cortex, but usually left unsutured. A piece of gelfilm is cut out and placed on top of the dura, and the bone is placed back. Usually it is not wired down, but merely fitted into its correct position. Histology in a successfully split monkey brain is shown in Figure 5.

The postoperative course is usually smooth and the animal more often than not is eating and drinking in normal fashion on the first postoperative day. Usually, the only noticeable effect of the surgery is the marked dilation of the pupils. In the cat it is noticeable, while

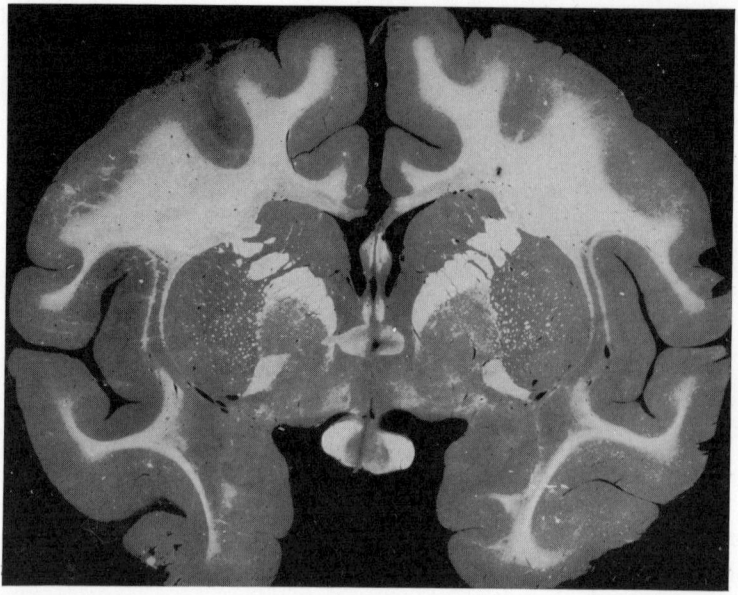

Figure 5. Cross-section of a monkey brain showing successful section of corpus callosum, anterior commissure, as well as midline section of the optic chiasm.

such dilation is variable in the monkey. This condition is produced by midline sectioning of the chiasm, and the reason for it is not entirely clear.

Behaviorally, cats and monkeys show severe impairment in stereoscopic vision as a result of the chiasm section. Cats, for example, will walk right off the end of the table in the first postoperative week; and monkeys, when placed in a large exercise cage, will walk about very gingerly and cautiously. This awkwardness in dealing with depth, however, is quickly compensated for at a gross level, and before long the animals are indistinguishable from normals. The stereoscopic defects remain, but must now be revealed through specific testing procedures.

The surgical procedure for the cat is much the same, the difference being that each step is more trying. The cat bleeds at every opportunity. Removing the bone in the monkey is a simple, bloodless maneuver, while in the cat it becomes a major effort necessitating bone wax and patience. The tissue itself is more fluid, less firm, and generally weak, making the use of pursuit and hunting probes more difficult. Bleeders occur more often, and like the bone, are less corrigible. Nevertheless, with a little experience one quickly masters the procedure and it becomes routine.

Lastly, to "split" the brain of the pigeon, only tectal and posterior commissures need be severed. Since all fibers cross in the optic chiasm, there is no need for surgical intervention here. The commissures rest above the midbrain and are immediately anterior to the base of the cerebellum. In preparation for the operation, the bird is anesthetized (Equi-Thesin) and shaved. The head is then placed in an appropriate stereotaxic apparatus. An incision approximately 1 inch long is made along the midline and the skin is drawn back to expose the skull. Since the skull is translucent, the central sinus can be seen quite readily. This landmark serves as the upper border of an opening approximately ½ cm square, which is to be drilled through the bone. Horizontal orientation is gained by placing the hole directly above the ear bars of the stereotaxic apparatus. Upon clearing the opening, the junction of the cerebrum and the cerebellum is revealed. The optic tectum is exposed by probing deep into the brain between these two bodies. However, considerable precaution must be taken at several points along the way. When approaching the final thin layer of skull, a very small burr must be used. All the white porous matter should be removed before attempting to cut through this thin encasement. It can be cut with dural scissors, and every care should be taken to keep the underlying dura intact. Otherwise, considerable bleeding can be expected, which may lead to irreversible brain damage. Once the brain is exposed, the dura along the juncture of the cerebrum and cerebellum is carefully slit. This can be done with the small gauge sucker described above. The same tool is used to gradually tease apart the cerebrum and cerebellum. With patience, the tectal commissures are eventually found at the base of this cleavage. It is easily severed with several brush strokes of the probing instrument.

Training Apparatus

The very nature of the split-brain preparation does not allow behavioral testing with standard equipment. Most operant conditioning setups are not equipped to limit the projection of visual information to one eye or the other. Similarly, the restriction of hand use is not easily possible. To meet these specific needs, several designs were worked up and tried for both the cat and the monkey.

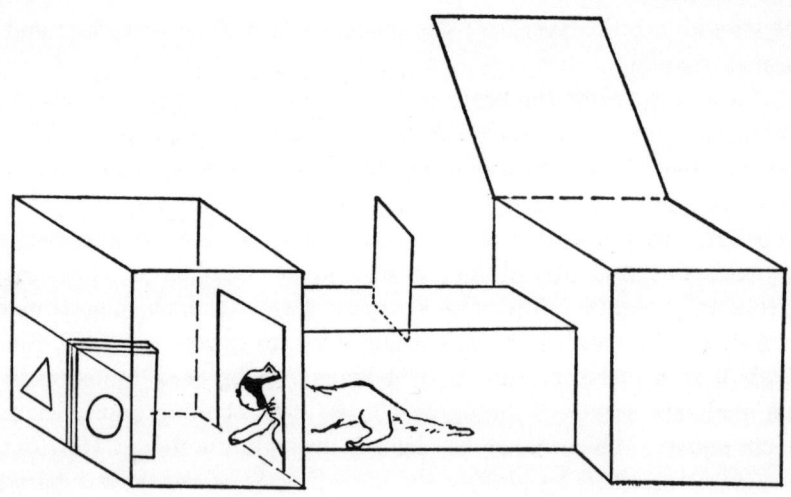

Figure 6. Cat-training box first used by Myers and Sperry. The animal is placed in the forechamber at the onset of each trial. An opaque door is then raised and the animal is free to choose one of two transparent doors, each with stimuli placed in them. A food reward appears outside the door behind the correct stimulus.

Operant techniques for the cat have never been extensively developed by psychologists, and as a result, in all the studies on split-brain cats to date, the same basic apparatus has been used; it was developed for that purpose, but necessitates hand training, with all of its problems. At the beginning of a trial, the animal is placed in the back of one of two chambers (Fig. 6). A door is raised, allowing entrance into an open chamber, where the animal is free to push one of two doors positioned side by side, each containing a stimulus display. Only the door with the correct stimulus affixed to it will open and give access to food, while response to the other door results in the sounding of a buzzer. At the end of the trial, the animal is physically removed from the front box and placed in the rear box. The stimulus patterns are changed on a pseudorandom basis; usually 25 trials per day are given. The visual input to one eye or the other is limited by means of a rubber mask.

It now seems that the apparatus described above is poor; any visual training procedure that does not eliminate the possibility of olfactory cues in training is poor at best. In the rat, the uncanny sophistication apparent for subtle discrimination is well known. The cat also is able to make such distinctions. Clear cues exist not only from the placement of the food reward itself, but also from the stimulus cards, which are continually interchanged from one side to the other. A simple remedy to these problems, of course, is to use stimuli projected onto translucent surfaces, and an odorless reward.

Perhaps a more serious fault in the basic design is the nature of the visual display itself. Horizontal arrangement of stimuli for an animal with a sectioned chiasm leads to needless additional troubles in interpretation of the data. Chiasm sectioning, of course, produces a binasal hemianopia, which in the cat reduces the overall visual capacity to about 35 percent of the normal level. This remaining capacity is then halved when one or the other eye is tested singly. In effect, each eye-hemisphere, when tested alone, sees but a fraction of the original scene, and then only that part of the visual field which is lateral to the vertical meridian. Accordingly, a stimulus falling outside of the remaining visual field might pass unnoticed in a discrimination task, thereby leaving a negative response open to a variety of interpretations.

Several investigators have tried to design a primate-testing apparatus that would fulfill all the requirements for split-brain testing and training. In the early days of split-brain research, attempts were made to use established training procedures and apparatus, such as the Wisconsin General Testing Apparatus. This led to difficult problems when attempts were made to restrict eye use or hand movement. In general, long-term eye use was controlled more readily than was short-term use by suturing one eyelid shut. When transfer tests were run on visual problems, the first eye was opened, and surgical closure of the other eye was performed. In retrospect, such procedures might well have precipitated a certain class of phenomena which become apparent only under such conditions.

Tactile discrimination training was carried out in a simple box that allowed access to the discriminanda with one or the other hand. This was usually accomplished with an adjustable sliding door that would allow a small hole to appear to the far right or left of the back panel near the side walls. Training and left-right alternation of the stimuli were carried out manually.

One of the first boxes specifically designed for testing split-brain monkeys was built by Trevarthen (Fig. 7). The main feature of his design was the introduction of polaroid techniques, allowing the simultaneous presentation of conflicting stimuli to each separate eye. That is, at a particular point in space, hemisphere I saw stimulus X, while hemisphere II saw stimulus Y. This testing method allowed for Trevarthen's studies on double-learning phenomena. Also, of course, his

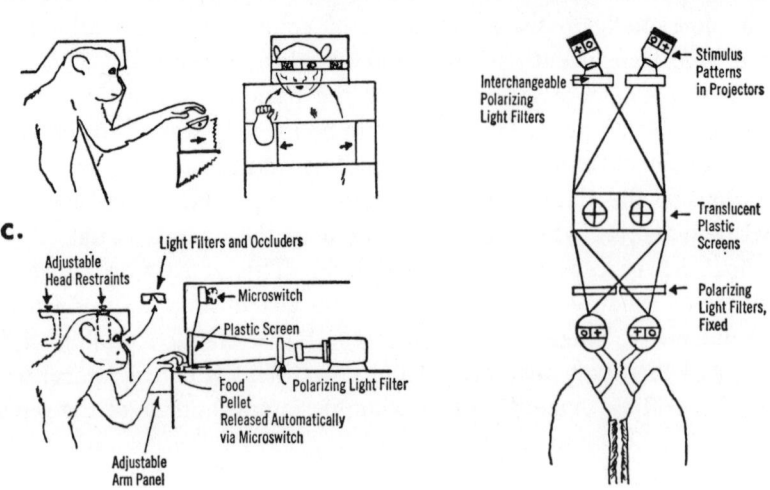

Figure 7. Behavioral training apparatus largely designed by Trevarthen. A. Profile and front diagrams of visual-discrimination training apparatus for controlling use of different eye-hand combinations. B. Diagram illustrating use of polarizing light filters to present different visual problems to right and left eyes simultaneously. Inversions produced by projector and ocular lenses are omitted. C. Profile sketch of same apparatus illustrated in B. (From Sperry, 1961)

apparatus allowed exclusion of either hand from response, as well as viewing by either eye, by covering the eye holes with opaque material. The disadvantages of this box include the necessity of manual training, and the problem of screen placement vis-a-vis horizontally placed stimuli. Again, as mentioned above, because of the nature of the visual-field deficits produced following chiasm sectioning, examination of the visual world through one eye causes much of the visual display to fall into the blind visual field. For example, fixation of the right panel by the left eye leaves the left panel in the blind field, and it is thus not available for visual comparisons. The animal must therefore learn to scan about when first exposed to visual stimuli in this kind of test situation. This learning procedure, however, might well effect some of the learning and transfer scores obtained from apparatus of this type.

A second design, largely a composite of boxes, independently developed by Sperry, Trevarthen, Hamilton, Mark, and myself (Fig. 8), allows for training in the animal's own cage, and all programming and recording is automated. During critical testing sessions, closed-circuit television monitoring is employed. This box is not without

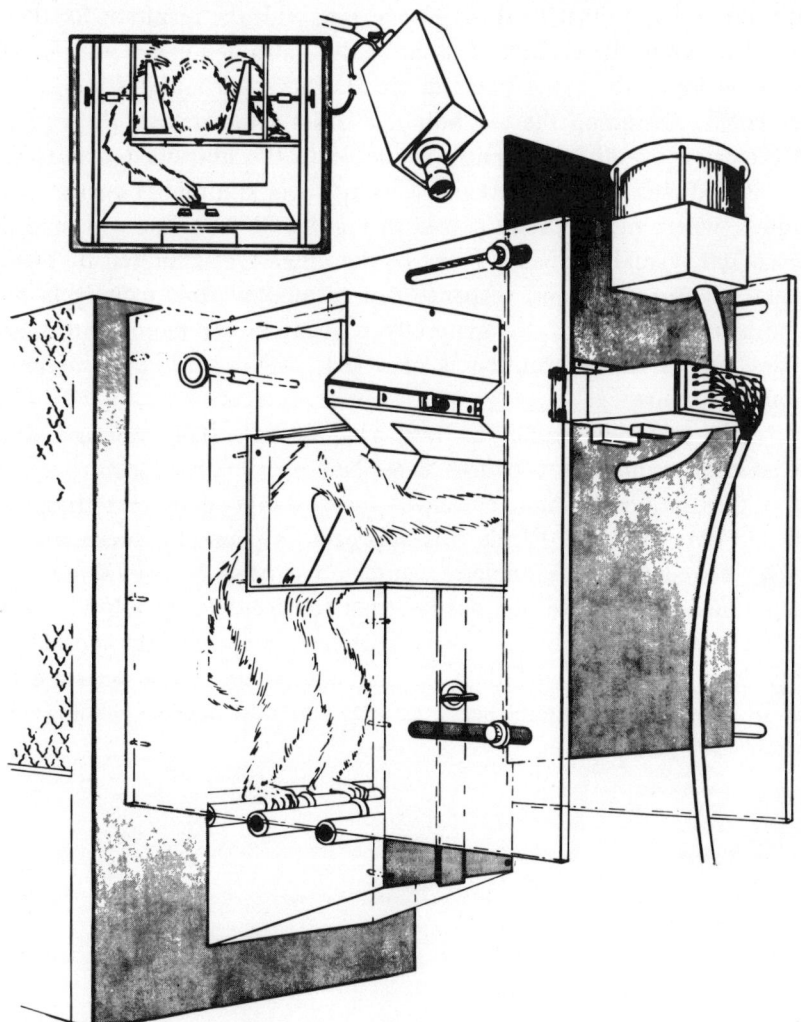

Figure 8. Sketch of automated testing apparatus. Compartment is attached to back of monkey's home cage and various adjustments permit selective control of eye and hand use. Knobs on each side control wedge plexiglass head restrainers and are easily adjusted for each animal. Television or motion-picture camera allows continuous nondisruptive observation.

problems, however, and in the main these problems center on the type of visual training usually carried out. The problem of visual-field deficit has been resolved in part by placing the response panels in a vertical plane. More recently, a "go/no go" discrimination has been employed, where the animals use only one response screen. Here, when learning a discrimination through one eye, with the resultant fixation of the stimulus in the midline, testing of the untrained eye would find the eye fixating at the exact point in space where the initial stimulus was presented. Assuming the test stimulus to be symmetrical, all necessary information would be instantly available to the untrained hemisphere.

Good success can be realized using more traditional operant techniques, where monkeys are placed in regular Skinner boxes. Using this procedure, visual exposure to one or the other eye is limited by opaque contact lenses and hand response can be limited (but usually is not). The opaque occluders are generally not left in for more than 1 or 2 hours, and if this precaution is observed, little or no inflammation or swelling occurs.

The stimulus display as well as data collection for most of the behavioral training procedures described above have been conducted with fixed-program logic systems, punched-tape data recording, and off-line data analysis. While this approach is generally successful, the emerging computer technology points up a need to re-evaluate these techniques. To be sure, the desire is not to do a 10-cent job with a 10-dollar machine. Rather the aim is to achieve more flexible and efficient experimental control and data-logging equipment. Once acquired and set in operation, it should serve an experimental neuropsychology laboratory for many years.

3

Sensory-Sensory Integration

One of the traditional approaches to studying brain function has been to produce punctate lesions in various cortical structures and to assess the resulting behavioral deficits, if any. In the early days of neuropsychology, it was thought that such neurologic insults would ultimately reveal the seat of various behavioral phenomena, such as learning and memory. Experiment after experiment was carried out, however, with no striking results forthcoming. Finally, Lashley (1950), wrote his classic paper on the matter, which among other things served notice that the brain-lesion approach was not going to generate the answers desired.

About this time, cybernetics and the related sciences appeared on the scene with the logical suggestion that the brain be viewed more as a dynamic system, with the parts interrelating in a most complex way to form the whole behavioral output. The idea was to emphasize systems analysis, not localization. More generally, the notion was that learning, memory, and the like, were more logical than topographic features of the brain system.

With the pendulum now swung way over in favor of the latter approach, the split-brain experiment gave new life to those who preferred to analyze brain functions with a knife. Instead of making massive lesions, discrete disconnections were possible. Or if the lesion approach was still favored by some, the split-brain allowed the experimental manipulation of only one hemisphere, thereby simultaneously halving the problem and also leaving one brain to the animal for maintenance of body functions. Additionally, the idea of the cortical island arose (Sperry, 1959). Instead of ablating the area to be studied, the split-brain allowed one to ablate everything in one hemisphere except the area under study, thus allowing for positive analysis of brain structures.

In the present chapter, recent experiments on sensory-sensory integration will be discussed and reviewed. Many of the experiments used the split only to simplify the surgical problem of producing bilateral lesions, while other studies examined the kinds of integration possible by both intra- and interhemispheric associated pathways. In particular, the studies involving tactual interactions will be emphasized more than studies on vision, with the latter being discussed in detail in Chapter 5, concerning the callosal code. Additionally, the recent experimental work on visual-tactual interactions will be discussed, as well as the interesting studies on visual-temporal disconnections.

Tactual Learning

Before the split-brain approach can be useful, the sensory input must be strictly lateralized. With vision, this is neatly accomplished by midline section of the optic chiasm. The central representation of tactile information, however, is less crisp. For example, somesthetic representation of the right upper extremity in the cat, monkey, and man is mainly contralateral. Some projections are also relayed ipsilaterally, with more representation apparent in the cat than the monkey, and in the monkey than man (Rose and Mountcastle, 1960).

Ipsilateral representation, however, is of a particular kind (Gazzaniga, 1968a). Generally, stereognostic information and the like from one paw is projected solely to the contralateral hemisphere. Ipsilateral information is of a more quantitative or less specific nature. Because of this, callosum-sectioned cats fail to show interpaw transfer of tactile discriminations (Stamm and Sperry, 1957). In contrast to the feline work, studies in the monkey have revealed variable results, with some reports claiming that intermanual transfer can occur in the callosum-sectioned monkey (Glickstein and Sperry, 1960; Ettlinger and Morton, 1966), while others claim it cannot (Ebner and Myers, 1962a). Also, Myers and Henson (1960) claim that no transfer occurs in the chimpanzee. In man, transfer is seen in some test situations (Gazzaniga et al., 1965).

These findings, at first, seem very puzzling, since the relative amount of ipsilateral information present is decreasing instead of increasing as one deals with more complicated nervous systems. It would not have been too surprising to discover that the relationship would be the other way—good transfer in the cat, with little or no transfer in monkey and man.

The data are critical for several reasons. Taken at face value, the data suggest that in monkey and man a subcallosal route is active in transmitting high-order tactile information. Alternatively, it could mean that both hemispheres learn a discrimination simultaneously—one via the contralateral system, and one via the ipsilateral system. Or, only one hemisphere learns the problem—but the opposite hand has access to the learning through the contralateral or ipsilateral system. Lastly, the data comment on the advisability of using the split-brain preparation to study sensory-sensory interaction phenomena, where tactile information is involved. If there is leakage of tactile information from one hemisphere to another, certain questions cannot be asked using the split. In the main, these would be aimed at teasing out the cortical and subcortical relationships in various learning phenomena.

There is a simple explanation for the existing experimental picture, that does not rely on the kind and amount of ipsilateral information present. Instead, it is proposed that the animal takes note of a variety of secondary cues, each of which can aid in the use of a basically psychologic strategy. The explanation is that monkey and man probably learn tactile discriminations in the contralateral hemisphere only. When the untrained hand is tested for transfer in the callosum-sectioned subject, the trained ipsilateral hemisphere can make use of enough cues available to it through the ipsilateral system to respond appropriately. Such features as height, weight, number of edges, length, and the like, are all features of a stimulus that the ipsilateral system can report (Gazzaniga, 1968a). In a highly trained discrimination, where use of one or two stimuli has been rewarded for hundreds, if not thousands, of trials, one of these parameters is likely to vary to a discriminable degree. As explained below in the section on intermodal transfer, this kind of mechanism is definitely present in man, and is presumably present in the monkey.

This notion makes several predictions about the data. In monkey and man, the transfer should sometimes be seen and sometimes not, depending on the ingenuity of the individual animal. That is to say, some animals might "figure out" the particular strategy, and some might not. Certainly the data support this notion, for there is an enormous variability in the amount of transfer seen in callosum-sectioned monkeys. In man, transfer is rarely seen if the above-described problems are taken into account. It is of interest to note that the absence of transfer in cats may reflect that they simply are not equipped to make use of such a complex strategy. Even simple instrumental conditioning is not transferable in the split-brain cat (Meikle and Sechzer, 1960).

The foregoing hypothesis would also suggest that the contralateral parietal cortex most likely would be involved in the memory process of tactual discriminations. Myers (1964) has shown that unilateral ablation of the contralateral hand area in the sensory cortex (area 3) leaves the monkey unable to perform a discrimination with the trained hand. Yet ablations of area 1 or 2, the associative cortex, yields no deficits. Once again, the baffling puzzle of where and, more importantly, how the engram is stored, eludes us. To observe that ablating area 3 produces deficits, only comments on the input circuit, yet an ablation one step beyond the primary input route yields no apparent behavioral deficits. To find the engram, which the split-brain technique limits to one-half of the brain, still remains the outstanding problem in neuropsychology.

Intermodal Association

The old problem of how stimuli presented in one modality can be identified in another has been examined extensively in the more specific context of determining how objects that are seen can be recognized through touch. Attempts at understanding the underlying neurology of this process in the monkey by producing ablations, and/or surgical disconnections between the relevant areas in the brain, have been largely frustrated because it has not yet been possible to establish a workable experimental situation where transfer between the two modalities consistently occurs. These data (Ettlinger, 1967) have been supported, and the implications from it extended in the recent reviews of Geschwind (1965a, b), who argues that such tasks are impossible because the monkey simply does not possess the necessary neurologic circuit. This notion is pivotal, of course, because the implications of such a view are serious and directive in terms of how one should proceed in studying neurocortical mechanisms of behavior.

Yet, the idea that animals are not capable of intermodal transfer strikes many as counterintuitive, at best. To explain high-order behavioral mechanisms with simple circuit diagrams seems to assume the question. Some data do exist for an alternative view, which in the main suggests that monkeys can perform intermodal associations. The study, outlined below, was carried out on two normal monkeys.

Using an automated testing device, each monkey learned two size discriminations (Fig. 9). Operation of the apparatus involved pull-

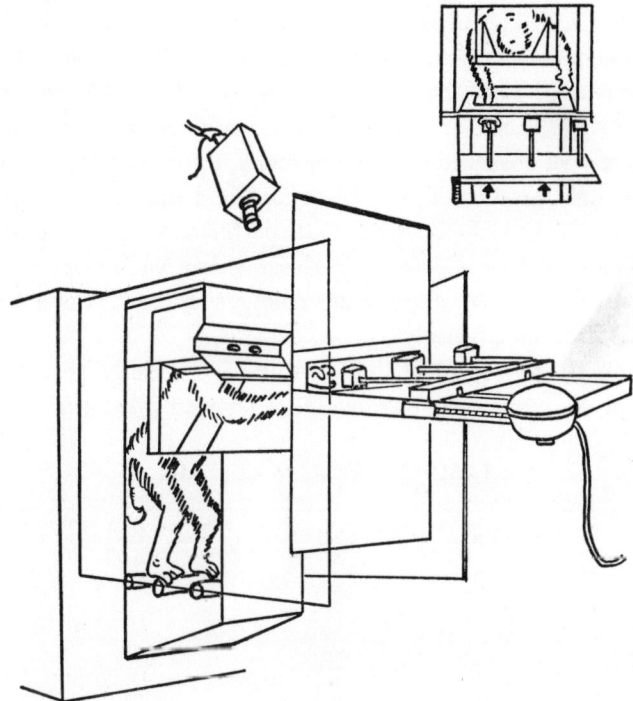

Figure 9. Automated visual-tactile testing device. S pulls one of two stimuli that are randomly alternated. After each trial, the manipulandum is automatically withdrawn out of sight and reach.

ing the correct one of two levers for a reward of a peanut delivered beneath the manipulanda. Right-left position of stimuli was randomized, and after each response the test objects were mechanically withdrawn from reach and view, followed by an intertrial interval of 10 seconds, and were then re-presented. In the first problem, the task was to distinguish between the larger of two squares, and in the second, the smaller of two spheres. One animal first learned the problem tactually, was then tested visually, and then learned the second problem in reverse order. The other animal first learned the problem visually, and was then tested tactually. All training was carried out in a well-lighted room under both modality conditions, with the exception that during visual training, two eye holes were opened up to allow the animal to view the stimuli. Possible auditory cues resulting from stimulus alternation procedures were randomized so as not to be a possible factor in mediating transfer. Also, it is important to emphasize that during the visual testing subsequent to tactual training, no intervening transparent screen or the like was used, in an effort to avoid letting the animal touch the object. The animal reached directly for the stimuli and the first one touched was counted as the response. Similarly, when visual training was used first, the animals manipulated the objects directly, as well as viewing them. In point of fact, with the aid of closed-circuit television, it was observed that the animals, upon learning the problem, always reached for the correct object first and did not make corrective movements, thereby suggesting that performance was under visual control. The objective of testing in this fashion was to opt for the best possible performance by minimizing changes in the test situation when shifting between modalities.

As can be seen from Table 1, there is virtually perfect transfer in three out of four cases. Animal DLY showed good transfer in both

TABLE 1. Trials to Criterion.

	Tactual	Visual	Tactual	Transfer
DLY				
Square	720	40		94%
Round		1280	120	90
EML				
Square		200	800	− 66
Round	480	0		100

directions, while animal EML showed transfer in only the tactual-visual test. When the problem was learned visually in this training procedure, it could be maintained that tactual learning was simultaneously occurring. When learning a task tactually first, followed by testing in the visual modality, this argument is ruled out, but replaced with the criticism that perhaps "one-trial learning" or the like took place. This, however, also seems unlikely in the light of the time taken to learn such problems at this stage of the animal's training experience.

Why high-level intersensory associations are seen here but not in other studies could be accounted for through several reasons, not the least of which is the nature of the training apparatus and procedure itself. In this box, the monkeys quickly learned how to play the game, and the actual motor responding was not changed or modified when the testing shift was made between modalities. In short, the transition between modalities was not severe or disruptive. This consideration is of clear importance even in visual-visual transfer tests. Monkeys, for example, can learn how to work a Wisconsin General Testing Apparatus and also a response-panel display system of the type described in Chapter 2. A plus/zero discrimination learned in one situation will not assist learning in the other, even when the actual stimuli are physically the same (Gazzaniga, unpublished). Lastly, the animals were learning what might be termed a principle and not a specific discrimination. What evidence there is for transfer in animals suggests that this would be the kind of problem that would show more intermodal transfer. These preliminary data, of course, are not so much offered as conclusive demonstration but as a gesture towards those who want to keep the door open on the question.

It is of special interest to study intermodal mechanisms in split-brain man, especially in the language-weak, disconnected right hemisphere. Results of these tests allow two main points. First, the nondominant, speechless, but semiverbal, right hemisphere is clearly capable of making high-order intersensory associations. Whether these match in extent and kind all those operations clearly present in the left, dominant hemisphere, has not been determined. In brief, the tests go something like this. (The procedure is described in more detail in Chapter 6.) Visual stimuli are quickly flashed into one or the other visual half-fields. If pictures are flashed into the left field, only the right hemisphere views the stimulus. Because these patients have had their cerebral commissures sectioned, the left hemisphere remains completely uninformed about the nature of the stimulus. Similarly, when stimuli

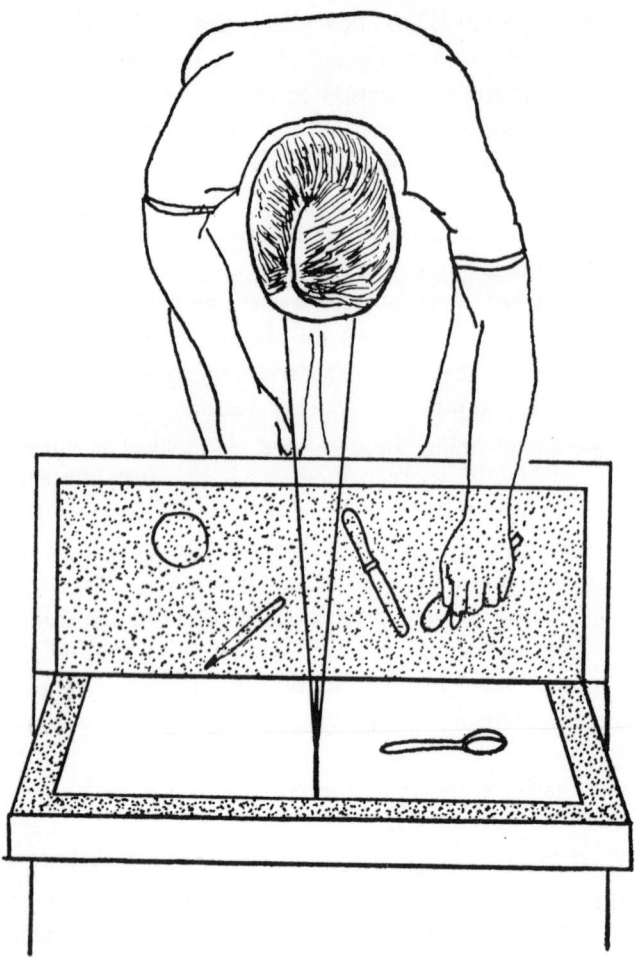

Figure 10. Visual-tactile association is performed by a split-brain patient. A picture of a spoon is flashed to the right hemisphere; with the left hand he retrieves a spoon from behind the screen. The touch information from the left hand projects mainly to the right hemisphere, but a weak "ipsilateral" component goes to the left hemisphere. This is usually not enough to enable him to say (using the left hemisphere) what he has picked up.

are flashed in the right visual field, only the left hemisphere is privy to the information.

The objects to be matched through touch are placed out of view, underneath the table, as shown in Figure 10. When the left hand is used, only the right hemisphere has access to the incoming stereognostic information. When the right hand palpates objects, only the left hemisphere is privy to the stereognostic information. (There are exceptions to these latter two statements, and they will be discussed below.)

Using this general testing procedure, stimuli were flashed to the right and to the left hemisphere, and tactual matches were subsequently requested with the appropriate hand. In all of the following tests, the left hemisphere proved capable of carrying out all operations requested. For example, when a picture of an orange was flashed to the left hemisphere, the subject would correctly retrieve with the right hand an orange from a series of objects presented out of view. The subject would then say in a normal fashion that the stimulus had been an orange. If the subject had used the left hand, with its major sensory projection going to the right hemisphere, and the visual stimuli were exclusively projected to the left hemisphere, intermodal associations would have failed. In order for an association of this kind to succeed in brain-bisected man, incoming visual and tactual information must be projected to the same hemisphere.

What is of more interest is that the speechless, nondominant, right hemisphere was also capable of making high-order intermodal matches. When visual stimuli such as triangles, ovals, squares, or pictures of objects such as pencils, spoons, apples, oranges, and so forth, were presented exclusively to the right hemisphere, the subjects would claim they saw nothing (i.e., the left hemisphere was talking), as it were—but then, with the left hand, they would retrieve the match from a series of objects. After each correct response, the subject was asked what had been retrieved. All replied they didn't know. Here again, it was the left hemisphere "talking," and it did not "know." It neither "saw" the visual stimulus nor had direct access to the tactual information. But because the right hemisphere performs consistently and well on such tests over a long period of time, it is assumed that it "knows" and is "aware" of the test stimulus: it isn't able to "talk" about it.

Again, because the visual information was exclusively flashed to the right hemisphere, the right hand (with its major sensory projections going to the left hemisphere) worked at only chance level.

Tactual-visual associations were also performed by each hemisphere. The subjects were first given something to palpate with either the left or the right hand, and were subsequently asked to point to a matching stimulus from a series placed in full view. All proved capable of doing this.

The conclusion from this sort of study is that as long as sensory and sensory-motor processes are featured in the same hemisphere, intermodal responses are possible not only in the dominant, language-strong, left hemisphere, but also in the disconnected, language-weak, right hemisphere. When the visual information is presented to one hemisphere and the tactual information to the other, no intermodal associations could be demonstrated. Further, in two patients who showed no linguistic competence whatsoever, intermodal matches were consistently performed at above chance level.

The second observation of interest to this discussion arises because some aspects of tactual information are projected to the ipsilateral as well as to the contralateral hemisphere (Fig. 11). That is, incoming tactual information is represented doubly—mostly in the contralateral hemisphere, but also weakly (and of a particular kind) in the ipsilateral hemisphere. Because this is the case, objects held in the left hand cannot be named, but the ipsilateral left hemisphere can describe certain features of the stimulus, such as whether it is there or not, and can therefore abstract stimulus parameters, such as "length" and "size" by how long a stimulus is present in the sensory field. The ipsilateral hemisphere notes the difference between deep and surface stimulation. By the expedient of pressing various aspects of the stimulus surface into the hand, it takes notice of such things as presence or absence of edges.

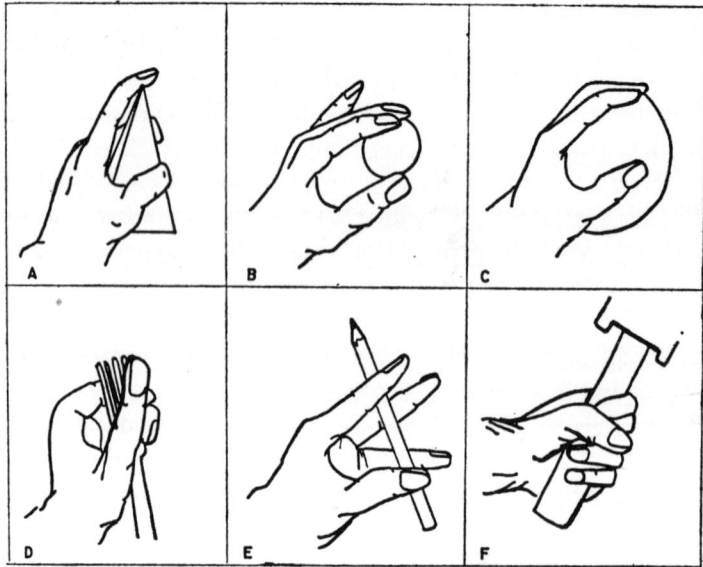

Figure 11. Illustration of different strategies employed by the left hand (ipsilateral) for detecting features of objects presented out of view.

Also, when thumping the hand along the object, the ipsilateral hemisphere can tell whether or not there are elevations in the object, and using this same trick, can count out various features of the object. Lastly, it can take note of how heavy the object is.

Clearly, if the subject is not "set," or if a limit is not put on what the stimulus might be, this information is usually not sufficient for correct identification of the object by the ipsilateral, left hemisphere. If, however, a clear limit is placed on what the objects might be that are presented to the left hand, then these cues are generally sufficient for correct recognition. For example, if the subject was told that either "a ball" or "a cube" would be available for palpation, a correct verbal report from the ipsilateral left hemisphere would be almost routine, for if the left hemisphere sensed the absence of edges in its exploration, it could deduce that the object must be a ball, not a cube. It appears, then, that these primitive features of an object, "leaked" to the left hemisphere, are sufficiently rich under the appropriate test condition to allow correct identification. These findings are of great interest, for they allow for speculation on what the brain is looking at during the identification of a tactual stimulus. Proper understanding of this aspect of the process would, of course, allow for a clearer understanding of why stimuli can be intermodally matched.

The foregoing observations indicate that linguistic competence is not a necessary condition for intermodal transfer. The combined data from the normal monkey and from the disconnected, language-weak, right hemisphere of man support this view. The implications of these findings are at least twofold. First, the pure connectionist view of mental processes is undercut in favor of a more liberal view, namely, that while circuitry is ultimately responsible for the underlying organization, it is hazardous to impress behavioral data on current-day knowledge of cortical circuitry. The failure to find association areas that receive rich connections from visual, tactile, and auditory areas in the monkey is of interest (Geschwind, 1965a, b), but now appears to have little or no correlation with intermodal transfer skills.

The second implication is that some kind of supramodal process is present. The nature of this system is still obscure, but hints of its organizational logic are seen in the analysis of the data obtained when the left hemisphere describes the quantitative nature of objects held in the left hand. In brief, this unique perceptual system allows consideration of what the brain may be taking note of in a particular stimulus display. The data suggest that a sensory system abstracts certain primitive features of the stimulus and commits these to a code, a rule mechanism, that all modalities have access to. In the context of the present problem, the implication would be that when the brain is set to attend to certain broad and universal features of a stimulus, then intermodal transfer occurs. If, on the other hand, it attends to only a "tactual" feature of the stimulus in a tactual-visual transfer test, or a "visual" aspect in a visual-tactual test, then no transfer would occur, because there would be no common information to the two systems. This kind of process would be present in animals and in illiterate humans. Once a system possesses the tools of language, however, it would most likely use them. Clearly, language greatly facilitates intermodal responses in man. On the other hand, a feature-abstracting system of this type may be the kind of information-handling system that is active prior to the linguistic encoding procedure in humans, and the engram type of information storage in both animals and man.

Visual-Temporal Interactions

The split-brain technique has been used extensively in studying the mysteries of infratemporal cortex. In brief, the hope was that crossed occipital-temporal lesions combined with differential sections of the corpus callosum would help clarify the role of cortical-cortical connections in visual-temporal interactions. This experimental approach, first used by Mishkin (1966) and Ettlinger (1959), has yielded results which strongly implicate cortical-cortical pathways working through preoccipital structures. The experiments were as follows. Visual input was limited to one hemisphere, with an infratemporal ablation in the same hemisphere, or placed in the visually deprived hemisphere. The channeling of the visual input to one side was accomplished through optic-tract sectioning, or through ablation of one of the occipital lobes.

If the corpus callosum remained intact, infratemporal lesions in the visually intact hemisphere resulted in far greater deficits than when the lesion appeared in the opposite, visually deprived hemisphere. In addition, if the posterior portion of the callosum was sectioned, in combination with the infratemporal lesion in the visually intact hemisphere, gross deficits were observed. These findings clearly suggest that the compensatory mechanism (active when visual information is limited to one hemisphere and the infratemporal mechanisms are limited to the other) takes place through the cortical-cortical connective system of the corpus callosum. This is consistent with a prior study, which in a preliminary way suggested an even more localized area within the callosum, namely, in the posterior half, anterior to the splenium (Gazzaniga, 1965).

In general, then, the major thrust of these findings is to argue for the view that a flow of information occurs from the primary visual areas into the infratemporal cortex for more extensive processing. This theoretical position and supportive evidence stands in marked contrast to the position of Pribram (1960) and his colleagues. They maintain that the infratemporal area has no direct connections with the visual occipital system, and that it is not an advance mechanism for visual analysis. Rather, it is their view that the infratemporal cortex acts on lower subcortical visual processes, and is able to modify and set the incoming visual information in a variety of ways. They liken the function to that of a "zoom lens"; that is, the infratemporal mechanism "zooms in" on the relevant information of a visual display, and pays particular attention to these features.

If this were indeed the mechanism and function of the infratemporal lobe, it would be hard to explain a great many of Ettlinger's and Mishkin's findings. For example, why would the split-brain animal with a unilateral infratemporal lesion be unable to perform discriminations readily with the lesioned hemisphere? If the mechanism of influence is downstream—subcortical and subcallosal—the intact infratemporal lobe on the other side ought to be able to assist the lesioned hemisphere. Pribram's hypothesis would have to take this possibility into account, and could, by further specifying that the infratemporal lobe functions only to modify the visual input of the homolateral visual field. This explanation, however, would not account for why cross-lesioned animals with the callosum intact can compensate. It follows that Pribram's notion would have equal difficulty explaining the partial callosal section work.

It is impossible to leave a discussion of this general topic without noting an interesting observation by Mishkin (1966), who found that with time the intact infratemporal cortex in a unilaterally lesioned animal can apparently induce the lesioned hemisphere to take on normal function. In brief, animals with an occipital lobectomy on one side, combined with an infratemporal lesion of the other, with much training were able to learn a visual discrimination. Upon subsequent section of the posterior callosum, the visually intact hemisphere, without an infratemporal cortex, was able to perform the discrimination! Yet, had the callosum been sectioned at the time of the lesion, no compensation would have resulted. This remarkable finding has been replicated by Reitz (1968).

The foregoing experiment comments on the boundary conditions of neural plasticity. It is not at all obvious that reorganization of this kind could take place in an adult primate. If one is committed to a rather pure nativistic view of brain circuitry, it would certainly appear the contribution of infratemporal cortex is not of a kind that requires special built-in circuits. It would appear to be a process that happens to locate during development in the infratemporal cortex. Additionally, whatever the nature of the central organizing forces, it would appear that they are no longer active in the adult brain. Rather, in order for compensation to occur, the instructions must be read out from an existing system.

4

Sensory-Motor Control Mechanisms

Any discussion of visual-motor coordination invariably leads one back to considerations of first causes in the nervous system. What acts upon what? How does a particular stimulus, say the plus of a plus/zero discrimination, precipitate and organize a visual-motor response to the exclusion of a multitude of other responses? Indeed, the question is complex enough in a more simple form—namely, how does a monkey manage to reach to a particular point in space? The issue has been studied extensively in the split-brain animal and in human patients with brain bisection. In this chapter the pertinent literature will be reviewed and discussed.

Following brain bisection, the question arises whether or not a particular hemisphere can guide and control the ipsilateral arm and hand as well as it can control the contralateral arm and hand. With the main motor-cortical controls for the right arm and leg located in the left hemisphere and those for the left limbs in the right hemisphere, section of the commissural cross-connections poses obvious problems for motor control and coordination, particularly where a performance triggered and directed from one hemisphere involves skilled movement in the distal extremities of the limbs represented in the opposite hemisphere. Does disconnection of the two cerebral hemispheres break a critical link in the interhemispheric sensory-motor sequencing of events resulting in impaired ipsilateral visual-motor coordination? Conversely, if no impairments are obvious, then it remains to be determined through what neurological systems, or by what psychologic strategies, the essential integration takes place.

Intrahemispheric Eye-Hand Combinations

There is general agreement that brain bisection has little or no effect on efficiency and accuracy of contralateral eye-hand combinations; studies in cat, monkey, and man all clearly show this to be the case. In the cat and monkey, one hemisphere can control the opposite extremity in visual-motor tasks.

In man, when stimuli were presented to one hemisphere, normal control over the opposite arm, hand, leg, and foot was observed. When a spot of light was flashed to any point in the right visual field, it could be pointed to accurately with the right hand, and when flashed in the left field, the left hand responded normally. Similarly, simple geometric shapes flashed to either field could be outlined or drawn correctly with the appropriate hand. Fine control of individual finger movements of the right hand was evident in tests involving blind manipulation of stimulated points on the fingers, and the mimicking of hand, thumb, and finger postures from sketches presented to the right-half visual field. If the stimuli were flashed to the left field, the left hand also performed accurately.

The effects of commissurotomy on ipsilateral eye-hand response, however, are complicated. To obtain a clear reading of the studies carried out to date, one must take into account a variety of factors, such as type of test used, age of animal, amount of head movement allowed, type of manual response recorded, amount of extra callosal brain damage present, and so forth; they are probably all critically involved.

Also, one cannot easily compare the results for cat with monkey, or monkey with man.

Interhemispheric Eye-Hand Combinations

Studies on the cat have not yet revealed any ipsilateral sensory-motor deficits. Both in discrimination learning (Schrier and Sperry, 1959) and in classical conditioning (Voneida and Sperry, 1961), the ipsilateral forepaw responds with the same accuracy, control, and efficiency as the contralateral paw. In many respects this is to be expected, especially when considered in the light of the studies of hemispherectomy and brain lesion in the cat. Following removal of the entire half-cerebrum, little or no impairment is observed in ambulation or in ipsilateral and contralateral eye-paw use (Bogen and Campbell, 1962). Similarly, removal of the frontal lobes bilaterally create no severe visual-motor problems (Voneida, 1967).

Reports on ipsilateral control in the monkey are many and varied. The first published studies were by Downer (1959), who claimed that following midline sectioning of the corpus callosum, anterior commissure, and optic chiasm, monkeys with vision limited to one eye (the other being stitched shut) were poor at guiding and controlling the ipsilateral arm. He reported the deficits to be severe, to the point that all animals neglected almost completely the ipsilateral arm. It did not matter whether the animal was involved in a learning situation or merely reaching for an object. Even when forced to use the ipsilateral arm by precluding movement with the contralateral arm, few, if any responses resulted.

These observations stand in marked contrast to a host of other reports. Myers et al. (1962), Gazzaniga (1964, 1966c), and Hamilton (1968), report that in simple reaching experiments the split-brain monkey works equally well with the ipsilateral and contralateral hand. If the animal is required to choose one of two visual stimuli in a discrimination situation, however, deficits in ipsilateral use have been observed (Gazzaniga, 1964; Trevarthen, 1962).

Before proceeding, it may be worthwhile to consider whether the reported difference between simple reaching movements and movements in a discrimination situation is real. At present, the answer is uncertain.

In all the reaching experiments, substantial control over the upper arm and shoulder would be adequate for accurate movements. Once these systems were set, the follow-through would result in hitting the target, even if the controlling hemisphere did not know the initial position of the wrist.

In the learning experiments reported to date, however, the animal has had to touch one of two panels—usually placed ½ inch apart in the horizontal plane. The testing box design was such that differential responses with respect to the panels would require control of wrist movement, as well as elbow and shoulder control. This might well explain the differences observed. In the reaching experiments, ipsilateral control must command only proximal muscles, whereas in the discrimination task, more discrete distal control is mandatory. In split-brain man, it is precisely this kind of control which is absent in the pure commissural lesion cases. It is entirely likely, therefore, that such deficits might be apparent in the monkey.

In addition to the foregoing, recent unpublished observations have shown that monkeys pressing one lever in a "go/no go" type of visual pattern discrimination show no ipsilateral deficits. Here, the animal was trained to hold down a lever for 2 seconds or longer for one stimulus in a discrimination pair and to release it within 0.5 second for the other discrimination. Animals trained contralaterally in the discrimination with one hand performed perfectly with the other (ipsilateral) hand. This rules out the suggestion that the differences observed are related to the presence of a discrimination per se (Gazzaniga, 1964).

Still left unexplained, however, are the enormous deficits reported by Downer (1959). The main difference in procedure was that Downer stitched one eye closed when testing for ipsilateral deficits. In the other reports, vision was occluded to one eye by mechanical devices present in the test chamber—and more recently by contact occluders. It might be argued that with Downer's technique of more or less chronic occlusion, attentional mechanisms became centered in the seeing hemisphere. The quick test procedures of others, however, might have left the two hemispheres in a more dynamic and cooperative state. This may be more likely than one might initially think. Several years ago, I designed an experiment to determine whether or not a split-brain monkey could attend to one or the other hemisphere at will, as it were. The animal learned a plus/zero discrimination in both hemispheres. Subsequently, using the polaroid technique developed by Trevarthen (1962), the problem was presented exclusively to the right eye in such a fashion that the plus was randomly correct half the time, and the zero half the time—that is, the problem was unsolvable. To the left eye, the discrimination remained the same as before, the plus remaining correct and the zero incorrect. Using this procedure, it could be concluded that only the left eye-hemisphere was attending if the score was 100 percent. If the score was lower, the animal was attending at least part of the time to the right eye. After extensive training over thousands of trials, the animal maintained a perfect score, thereby indicating that only the information projected to the left hemisphere was being processed. Although freehand use was available to the animal, the contralateral right hand was always used in response.

At this time in the training history, when the animal was forced to use the ipsilateral left arm, an awkwardness of reach was observed, the animal sometimes missing the button by 2 to 3 inches. In addition, the animal perseverated in the incorrect response, and the arm flopped about in an abnormal fashion. From this, one could argue that the attentional processes had been conditioned to be centered in one hemisphere, and when ipsilateral eye-hand combinations were called in, one saw the abnormal reaction paralleling that described by Downer.

Of course, a more parsimonious explanation of Downer's results is that during the early days of split-brain surgery, significant amounts of extracallosal brain damage were accidentally produced in the course of the surgical procedures. This correlation has been made in our own colony, and now that surgical techniques are sufficiently developed, one can experimentally produce ipsilateral deficits by poking and sucking here and there during the course of the operation.

Eye-hand control has also been studied in the chimpanzee (Black and Myers, 1964, 1965). In simple reaching tasks, the split-brain chimpanzee has little or no problem in carrying out accurate responses with the ipsilateral or contralateral hand. These findings are consistent with work on cats, monkey, and man. The authors maintain, however, that ipsilateral deficits can be elicited and are quite striking in more complex tasks that require "gnostic sophistication." Curiously, the task used in the experiment was a latch box problem—a task that requires no visual control for solution. Yet, the authors maintain that the problem was a visual-motor problem, and conclude that because there is poor intermanual transfer on the task, it reflects a problem of visual-motor control! Clearly, the animals had learned the problem tactually, and had not performed the problem well with the untrained hand because of the lack of interhemispheric transfer following split-brain surgery for tactual discriminations of this kind. Consistent with this interpretation is their observation that complete "transfer" occurred to the untrained eye if the trained hand was used in response. In view of the multitude of studies on the lack of transfer of visual tasks following brain bisection, how could this problem be looked upon as a visual

MOTOR RESPONSES TO VERBAL COMMANDS

CASE I:

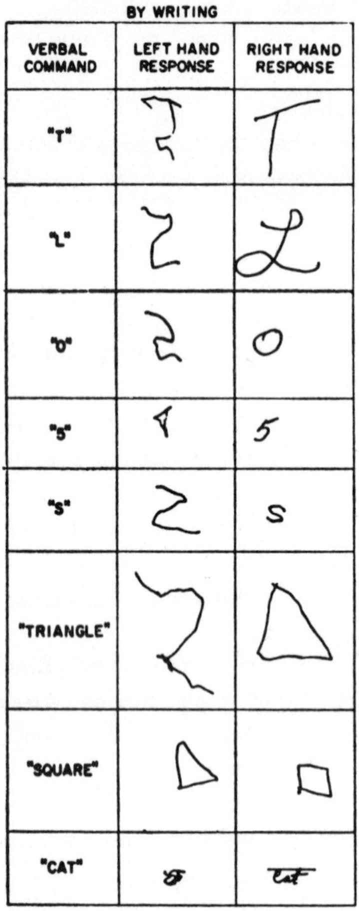

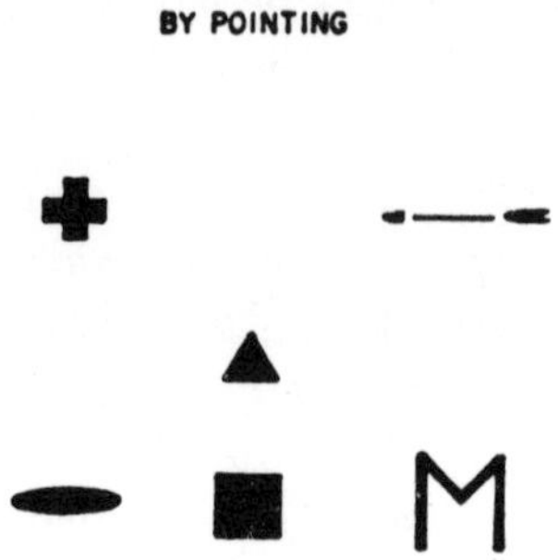

BY WRITING

VERBAL COMMAND	LEFT HAND RESPONSE	RIGHT HAND RESPONSE
"T"	⌐	T
"L"	∠	ℒ
"O"	⌐	O
"5"	ʡ	5
"S"	∠	S
"TRIANGLE"	(scribble)	△
"SQUARE"	◇	▱
"CAT"	✗	cat

BY POINTING

+ — ◂
▲
— ■ M

SUBJECT REQUIRED TO POINT TO A REQUESTED FIGURE
a) For wrist movement, actual size of response pattern sheet was 8 1/2 × 11"
b) For shoulder movement, actual size was 22 × 28"

CASE I: 2 3/4 YEARS POST-OP
RESULTS

Right Shoulder	Right Wrist	Left Shoulder	Left Wrist
21	21	15	3

Scores refer to number of correct responses in 21 trials. (Chance = 3)

Figure 12. Case I of the series displayed a marked apraxia with the left arm. Responses requiring control of more distal musculatures were particularly disturbed. When directed to write a series of letters or words with the right arm, there was little or no problem. Meaningful responses with the left hand, however, were not possible. In tests that required only gross control of the left arm involving mostly proximal muscles, good control was evident. In further analysis, the left-side apraxia was shown to be a product of the extracallosal damage present in this patient (see text).

task? Nonetheless, the results are discussed in these terms, and the authors propose that subcortical mechanisms are active in the simple reaching experiments while the latch box problem suggests that more cortical mechanisms are active. It seems fair to say that the experimental results hardly justify such reasoning; the more general question of eye-hand control in the champanzee has been examined in visual reaching experiments only.

In man, the degree of ipsilateral deficit observed following lesion of the corpus callosum is still debated. Geschwind (1965a, b), in a recent review, asserts that lesion of the callosum produces a severe, left, ideomotor apraxia. Normal right-handed patients with the left hemisphere dominant for speech and language are, in response to verbal command, unable to make purposeful movements with the left hand. In all the lesion cases he reports and reviews, as well as our first case of surgical disconnection of the cerebral hemispheres, the patients, in addition to their partial or complete callosal lesions, had considerable extracallosal damage. This has proved to be a critical factor in the degree to which a disconnected hemisphere can guide and control the ipsilateral hand and arm (Fig. 12).

Only recently has it been possible in man to critically analyze the role of the corpus callosum in interhemispheric visual-motor integration. The majority of the previous reports are simply uninterpretable because of the unknown amount of extracallosal damage present. In the more recent series of cases, several of the patients were relatively free of extracallosal brain damage. Two of the patients that were carefully studied had rapid recovery from surgery and were selected for extensive study as being representative of pure lesions of the commissures. The overall picture of apraxic disturbances in these selected cases was mild. Except for fine differential movements of thumb and fingers, each hemisphere appeared to exert good control over movements of the ipsilateral as well as the contralateral limbs (Fig. 13). Pronounced deficiencies were evident with lateralized visual input in tasks where the right hand had to be directed from the right hemisphere and the left hand had to be directed from the left hemisphere.

In brief, when the left hemisphere attempted to control the left subordinate hand, performance went well as long as the response could be carried off without specific control over the distal musculature. Thus, the patients could readily point to an object in the left visual field and could trace or draw its outline either in the original position in which it was seen, or on a piece of paper. When single printed

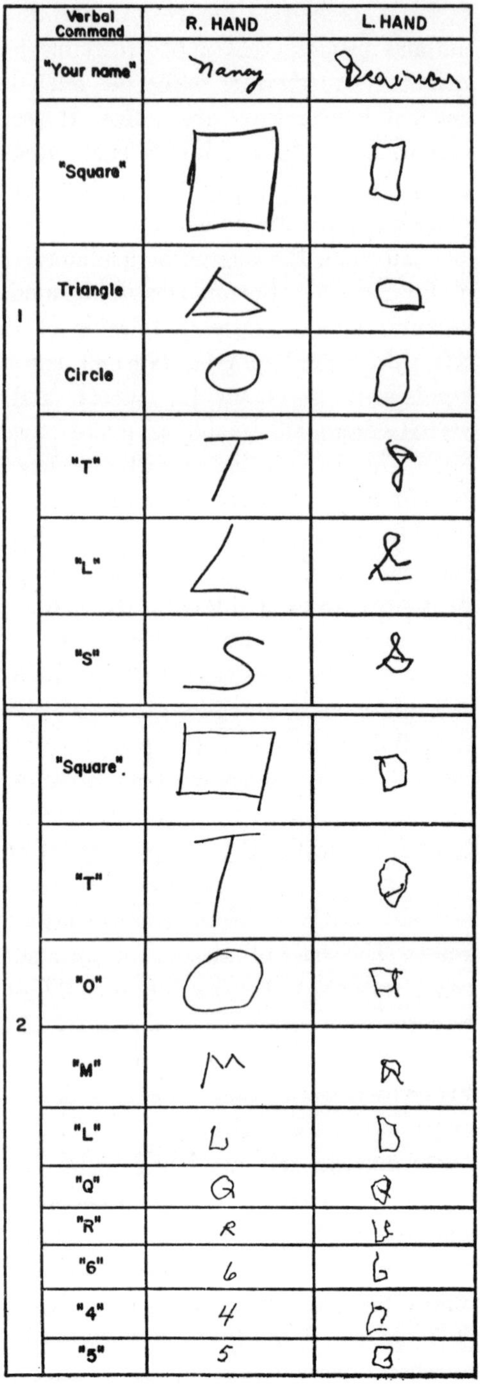

Figure 13. Motor responses to verbal commands in Case II. The results more closely resemble the course of recovery for the pure commissural lesion class. While she had considerably more problems than did Case III, the above shows how her performance cleared up with good control of left hand by the left language hemisphere at six to eight months. The column at the left of each section indicates postoperative month in which written responses were recorded.

	Verbal Command	R. HAND		L. HAND
4	"If I went to the store I would buy a toy."	*If I went to the store I would buy a toy.*		
		L. HAND	Example Printed	L. HAND COPY
		♂ ⊤ ▷ ∩ ∘	BOY	BOY
		Tea +	CAT	CAT

	Verbal Command	R. HAND	L. HAND
6	"This is a pretty day"	*This is a pretty day*	*(scribble)*
	"Your name"	*Nancy*	*No No~*
	"Square"	▱	▱
	"Circle"	○	⟁
	"Triangle"	△	△
8	"Comb"	*Comb*	*(scribble)*
	"spoon"	*Spoon*	*Spoor*
	"cat"	*Cat*	*Cat*
	"Your name"	*Nancy*	*Nancy*
	"Your Husbands name"	*Bud*	*Bud*

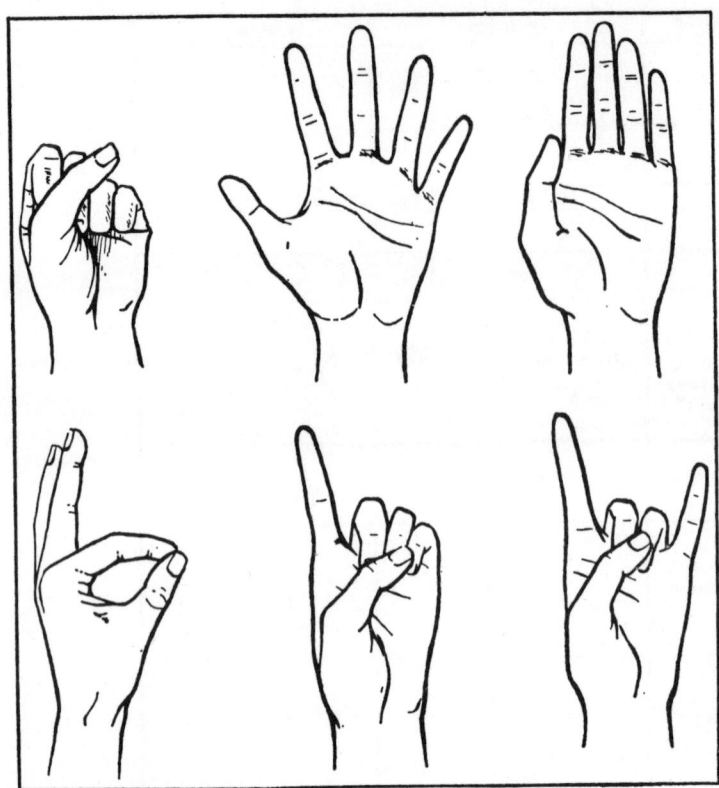

Figure 14. Sample drawings of different hand positions that were flashed to left or right hemisphere to test ability of each half brain to execute control over ipsilateral or contralateral hand.

words were flashed tachistoscopically to the left hemisphere, they could generally be written out with the left hand, and the same was true for word or number answers to verbal or arithmetic problems presented orally. Ipsilateral control from the dominant hemisphere appeared at its worst in tasks in which the left hemisphere was required to direct the individual fingers of the ipsilateral hand (Fig. 14). For example, when outlines of the hand and fingers held in a variety of postures were flashed to the major hemisphere the patients readily mimicked the posture with the contralateral right hand, but usually failed with the left hand. Correct responses were obtained with the left hand, only when it was mimicking the simple postures such as making a fist or extending all digits at once. The same postures and movements required in the above test could be performed by the left hand when the cortical control was shifted to the right hemisphere by presenting the sensory stimulus to the left-half visual field or the left hand.

The greatest impairment detected with nonverbal testing was seen in tests in which the minor, right hemisphere was called upon to control movement of the right hand. Good performance was obtained in tests that involved simple direct response like pointing to an object or tracing the outline of something flashed to the left visual field. Responses of this kind involved shoulder movements mainly. At times the patients could also draw correctly with the right hand various simple geometric shapes presented to the left-half visual field, or the left hand when the latter was out of sight. However, the results were erratic, and failures were common. To what extent the poor performance of these latter tests reflected an inadequate control system from the right hemisphere to the motor centers involving the digits is not certain. Often one gained the impression that the difficulty lay in the competition for right hand control that was continually and regularly coming from the major hemisphere.

In summary then, ipsilateral control is good in brain-bisected man so long as one does not call into action the most distal musculatures of each limb. In the brain-bisected cat, monkey, and chimpanzee a disconnected hemisphere can accurately guide and control the ipsilateral limb. Performance breaks down when the response requires discrete control of the most distal musculatures. In the monkey, while there have been conflicting reports, reconciliation is possible following close examination of the experimental situation used.

The question becomes, therefore: What is the neurologic organization underlying this ability of one hemisphere to accurately control the ipsilateral limb? The problem has been attacked experimentally in the monkey by myself and others; the following is a review of some of the mechanisms that have been proposed to explain this phenomenon.

One of the most frustrating aspects of studying ipsilateral eye-hand use in split-brain animals is in knowing that there are probably several mechanisms the animal makes use of, and it is likely that the animal could perform adequately using any one of them. Just when the experimenter thinks one mechanism has been isolated, the animal shifts to another mechanism, leaving the hypothesis confounded. Nonetheless, this is one of the most intriguing problems in research on visual-motor coordination, and the potential rewards are worth the continuing setbacks. The overall attractiveness of the problem lies in the simplicity and the clarity of the ever-present question—namely: How does one disconnected cerebral hemisphere guide and control the ipsilateral hand? A clue to the essential integration here may yield important insights to the general problem of visual-motor integration.

Role of Subcallosal Interhemispheric Connections

In addition to the commissures routinely sectioned in the split-brain operation, there are several others. The principle remaining interhemispheric systems are the posterior commissure, the habenular commissure, the commissures of the superior and inferior colliculi, and the interthalamic commissure. There are several other still lesser commissures, such as Maynert's, Gudden's, Forel's, and so forth. In addition to these structures, the hemispheres can also intermix information in the reticular formations of the upper and lower brain stem. In other words, there are several pathways through which an ipsilateral visual-motor response could be mediated. This notion has been directly tested in the monkey by carrying out deep-split surgery in the midline, down into the medulla (Fig. 15).

These animals showed cerebellar signs; they suffered from a marked asthenia in the hind limbs and all showed some ataxia when reaching. Assymmetrical facial paralysis was usually present, and was presumably due to swelling or midline bruising, or both. With both eyes open, conjugate eye movements were observed only occasionally. Usually, the eyes appeared to be moving independently, and no discernible pattern was observed. Nonetheless, the animals using one eye, the other being occluded, could at times momentarily fixate on an object. After approximately three to four weeks of intensive postoperative care, the animals recovered to a large degree, except for some eyelid droop. Clear signs of postural imbalance, ataxia, and ocular motor deficiencies remained.

Despite all of the foregoing abnormalities, it was clear that the animals with deep midline surgery could perform ipsilateral eye-hand responses. They were able to reach out in the correct direction to retrieve grapes placed anywhere in the visual field. In making these observations, however, one had to exclude from consideration blind, sweeping movements of the hand, which appeared not to be triggered in response to a discrete visual target. Accuracy of response was far

SENSORY-MOTOR CONTROL MECHANISMS 45

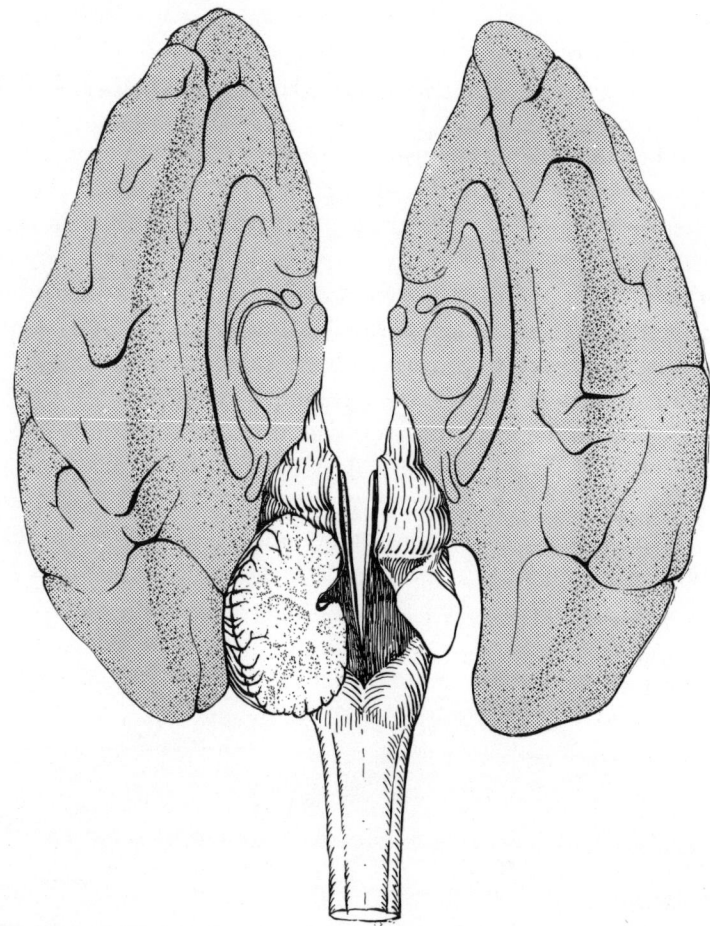

Figure 15. Deep midline surgery was extended down to include medulla in four monkeys. All animals proved capable of performing visual-motor tasks with ipsilateral eye-hand combinations.

better in the second to fourth months after surgery than in the first. Slight errors were frequently made in reaching, such that the animal might miss the object by an inch or so on either a horizontal or vertical plane. However, their response was always in the right direction, and was rarely grossly in error. There appeared to be little appreciation of depth. It was as if only cues on the horizontal and vertical axis were used. Once these were noted, the hand reached out blindly until it hit the object, whereupon tactual systems initiated the appropriate hand movements for retrieving the food morsel.

Role of Direct Ipsilateral Fibers

Another possible mechanism active in the execution of ipsilateral eye-hand responses is that the arm or limb ipsilateral to the seeing hemisphere may be directly controlled by fibers originating in the ipsilateral hemisphere. Analysis of this notion breaks down into three categories: (1) Is the fiber system sufficiently strong to carry out the control in the absence of the contralateral motor system? (2) Does the ipsilateral system work in concert with the contralateral system? (3) Is the ipsilateral system part of the pyramidal system?

In answer to the first two questions, it would seem quite clear that if an ipsilateral system is active it does not possess sufficient power to control movement in the absence of the tonic effects of the contralateral motor system. Hemispherectomy studies clearly show that the remaining hemisphere is, at best, poor in guiding the paralyzed hand (While et al., 1959). Likewise, studies in split-brain monkeys have

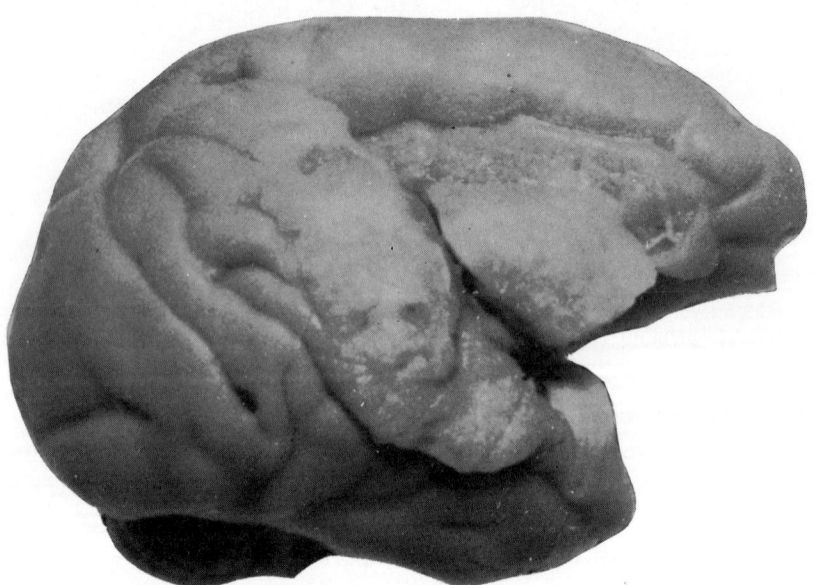

Figure 16. Brain of a monkey showing extent of cortical lesion that does not interfere with ipsilateral eye-hand control when leisoned hemisphere attempts to control the ipsilateral hand. The animals in both free reaching situation as well as in discrimination learning show no major problems in ipsilateral control.

shown that when a particular hemisphere is damaged even to a slight degree the opposite hemisphere is poor at carrying out ipsilateral tasks (Gazzaniga, 1966c). It would seem, from these and other studies, that if ipsilateral motor systems were critically involved in these kinds of eye-hand response, then they would be effective only when the integrity of the contralateral motor system is assured.

Assuming for the moment that such a mechanism is active, the question arises: What is the neurologic nature of the ipsilateral control? At present there are little direct data on the issue, the evidence to date suggesting that the pyramidal system is not crucially involved. Removal of the entire frontal lobe and part of the parietal lobe does not eliminate good control from the lesioned hemisphere (Fig. 16). While the pyramidal tract does not solely originate in the pre-and postcentral cortex, the great majority of its fibers originate in these areas. Conclusive demonstration that such control is not active would involve sectioning the tract unilaterally at the medullary level. This notion of bihemispheric control cannot be definitely eliminated as a major mechanism involved in ipsilateral control. The following experiments, however, present certain difficulties for this view.

Target Information Carry-Over Through Cross-Cuing

A third strategy likely to be employed by the split-brain animal in making ipsilateral eye-hand responses is what I have called the "cross-cuing" mechanism (Gazzaniga, 1966c). The general notion here is that hemisphere A can set up hemisphere B to make a correct response through a variety of ways, but each way requires that hemisphere B act in response to a cue made available to it in the peripheral apparatus by hemisphere A. The cross-over of information is not through the central neural channels; instead, it is by one hemisphere taking note of cues made available to it by the overt bodily-systemic changes executed by the other hemisphere. A similar notion has been proposed by Mark and Sperry (1968) for bimanual coordination tasks involving somatosensory cues.

The original observation that suggested this hypothesis was as follows: Several split-brain monkeys with a variety of lesions and midline disconnections were filmed in slow motion while retrieving food morsels presented about them. In general, one eye was occluded with an opaque contact lens and the ipsilateral hand was restrained. This left the animal free to use one hand and to view the world through only the ipsilateral eye. Gross observation in this kind of task, without the aid of slow-motion cinematography, suggested no mechanism whereby the animals were successfully carrying out ipsilateral eye-hand responses. The movements were too quick and crisp for teasing out the possible strategies used.

Reviewing these same movements on slow-motion film, where time for observation for a single movement is greatly expanded, revealed the strategy used. When a food morsel was held out in a particular part of the visual field, the animal would scan the visual world until the object came into view. Then, it would fixate the object, orienting to it with eye, head, and neck movements—all following into line. The animal would then reach out with the ipsilateral arm to the relevant point in space; several animals actually closed their eyes during the reaching movement itself!

This observation supports the cross-cuing notion. The seeing hemisphere takes note of the point in space to be obtained, fixates on the point, thereby allowing the nonseeing hemisphere all the information it needs to carry off a motor response because of the nonseeing hemisphere's ability to read off eye, head, and neck position by means of nonvisual proprioceptive systems. With this information input held at a constant level, the blind hemisphere can either itself decide to reach to the point in space, using the readily controllable contralateral arm; or the seeing hemisphere, by some kind of peripheral jerk or grunt, or the like, could signal the blind hemisphere to go when ready.

At this point, it is of interest to take stock of how much this scheme might explain. To begin with, the utilization of cross-cuing information would enable a split of any depth, with or without massive lesions in one hemisphere, to carry off ipsilateral movements with little defect—as is the case. No matter how much the central neurologic state is altered or destroyed, the animal has ways of "jumping" the split, or "skirting around" the effects of the lesion through these cross-cuing mechanisms. To eliminate surgically the kind of information exchanged would be exceedingly difficult, if not impossible.

The poor ipsilateral control seen in discrimination learning can also be explained. In the studies to date, all animals were tested for their general ability to retrieve food morsels using ipsilateral control under conditions of no head restraint, and no deficits were observed. When deficits were observed, the animals were attempting to hit one of two buttons placed laterally to each other, their heads being completely restrained, thus eliminating any bodily orientation to the stimulus. In this situation, the proprioceptive feedback would be minimal. Up to this point, the theory correctly explains why the animals experience some difficulty in carrying off ipsilateral eye-hand responses.

The foregoing observations and analysis lead to experimentally testable problems. In general, careful measurements of eye-hand accuracy in the normal and split-brain animal under conditions where the head is both restrained and unrestrained, combined with restriction of eye and hand use, ought to yield clear differences in performance related to the amount and type of proprioceptive feedback from eye, hand, and neck. The following discussion concerns a series of experiments aimed at teasing out these various considerations.

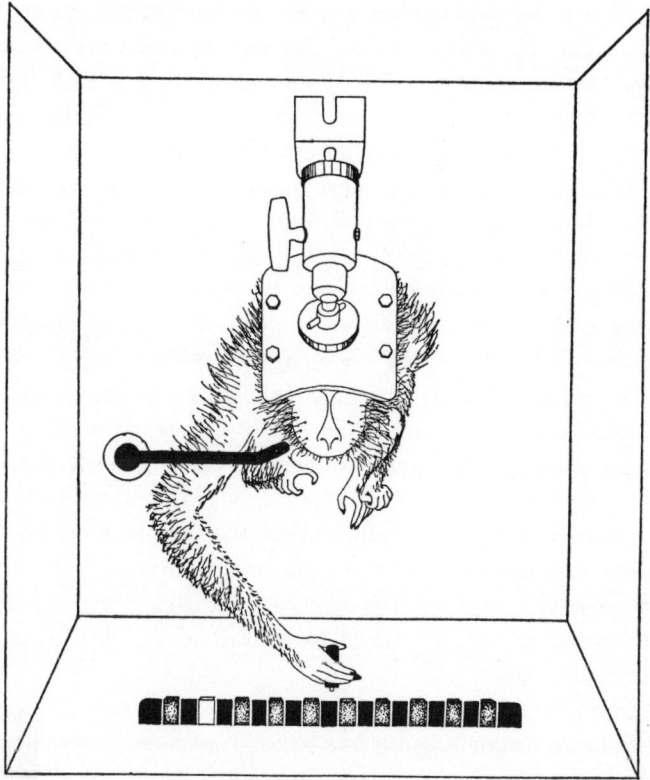

Figure 17. Automated testing device for measuring accuracy of reaching. Liquid reinforcement is delivered through solenoid drinking tube to right of animal. Lever below response buttons activates trial.

The apparatus, especially designed for the experiment, consisted of 10 response levers, ⅜ inch wide, spaced 1½ inches apart on center (Fig. 17). The animal's head was fixed straight ahead, with the midline falling between levers 5 and 6. Between each lever was placed a solid divider, which in effect required the animal to make individual finger movements in order to hit in between the dividers placed on each side of each lever.

Directly beneath the series of response levers and in the midline was another lever, which was used by the animal to initiate the trial. Triggering this lever resulted in illumination of one of ten lights arranged on a horizontal scale, as illustrated in Figure 18. Coincidence of stimulus position and response choice commands a grape juice dispenser to reinforce the subject.

Restraining head movements involved implanting four stainless steel machine screws (¾ inch, 6–32)—two on each side on the midline of the skull (Evarts, 1968). The two screws were reinforced by including between them a stainless steel separating bar. A lightweight but sturdy aluminum hat was fitted onto the four protruding bolts, with a hole in the center, tapped to accept the screw connector of a universal Leitz ball-and-socket camera mount. With the ball-and-socket joint loose, free head movements were easily possible; but with the joint fixed, no head movements were possible, leaving the animal free to make only eye movements.

Three control animals (BNE, unoperated; CLN, callosum sectioned, chiasm intact; and NTW, chiasm sectioned, callosum partially sectioned) performed with accuracy and good control in all eye-hand combinations, with the head either held or free (Fig. 18). NTW's performance dropped off in the blind half-field of each eye, but this reflected a sensory deficit more than a visual-motor inadequacy. In general, as long as sensory information was available to each hemisphere either through the callosum, the uncut chiasm, or both, no deficits were observed in the tests used. In the following, therefore, the deficits recorded are not a product or artifact of the test procedure and apparatus themselves.

With no restrictions on visual input or restraint of head movement, split-brain animals using one hand were able to reach accurately with little or no practice to all levers on the horizontal scale (Fig. 19). With the head fixed, only minor difficulties were seen.

Contralateral eye-hand pairing revealed only a slightly different picture. With the head free, good performance was elicited for lights falling into the intact visual field, and with little or no practice, responses became accurate in the blind field. In carrying out these latter responses, each animal would characteristically scan the response panel until catching sight of the illuminated level and then, orienting towards it, would respond. With the head fixed, the responses in the intact visual field remained good, whereas the accuracy of responses in the blind half-field dropped off. In the animals that were allowed additional blocks of trials, the score improved for the stimuli falling into the blind field. Close observation of the animals' behavior under these conditions revealed that scanning movements of the eyes were frequent. Upon seeing the stimulus, they would hold the eyes fixed until making the response. All responses made with the contralateral eye-hand pair appeared crisp and directed, with good control of hand movement evident.

The most severe deficits were observed with ipsilateral eye-hand combinations. With head free, ipsilateral responses were relatively good in the visual half-field, but generally decreased in accuracy in the blind field. With practice, responses in the blind field improved markedly. Again, direct observation of the animals' responses during these trials showed that they scanned the board until the illuminated lever came into view, and then fixated on it during the response. With the head restrained, large deficits were seen when both the intact and the blind visual field were used, the accuracy improving with practice. Generally, using this eye-hand combination proved disturbing for the animals; all took longer to respond, became agitated, and generally awkward in their response.

With the head free or restrained, a striking feature of the response was the awkwardness of hand movement. Instead of striking a lever with precision and tone, as seen with the contralateral eye-hand pair, the response (with respect to the hand, not the arm) took on a blind, groping posture, with the fingers widely separated. Only with effort, and usually some practice, could the animal control the hand sufficiently well to depress one of the levers in between the two side guards.

Several trends are clearly apparent. First, the experimental group performed consistently better when their heads were free. The degree of impairment produced by restraining the head progressed, as more stringent visual restraints were imposed. These findings are consistent with the view that head position is contributing to overall accuracy of

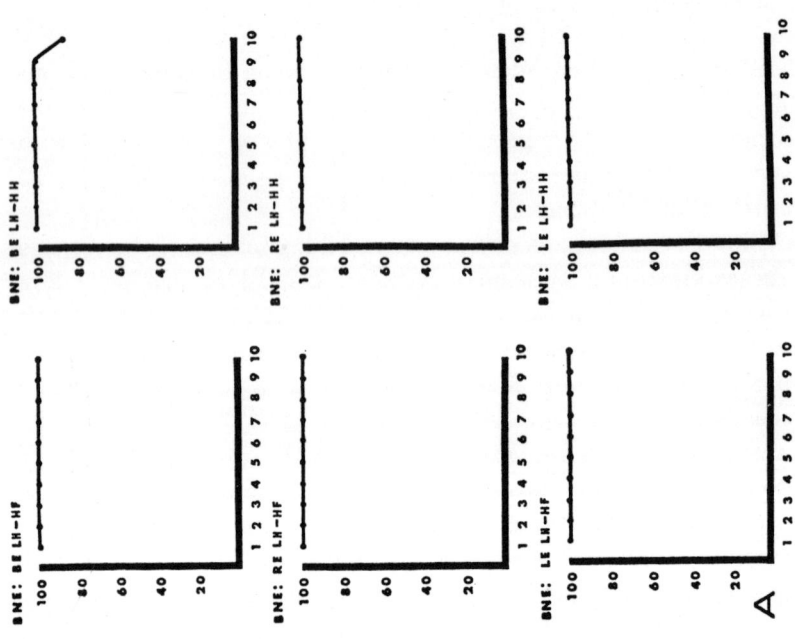
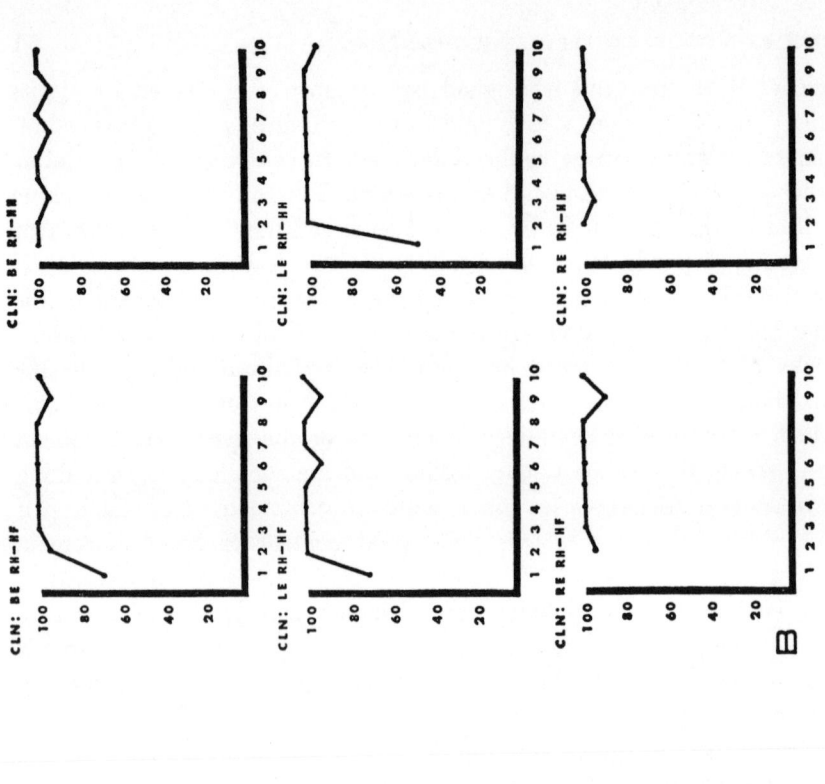

52

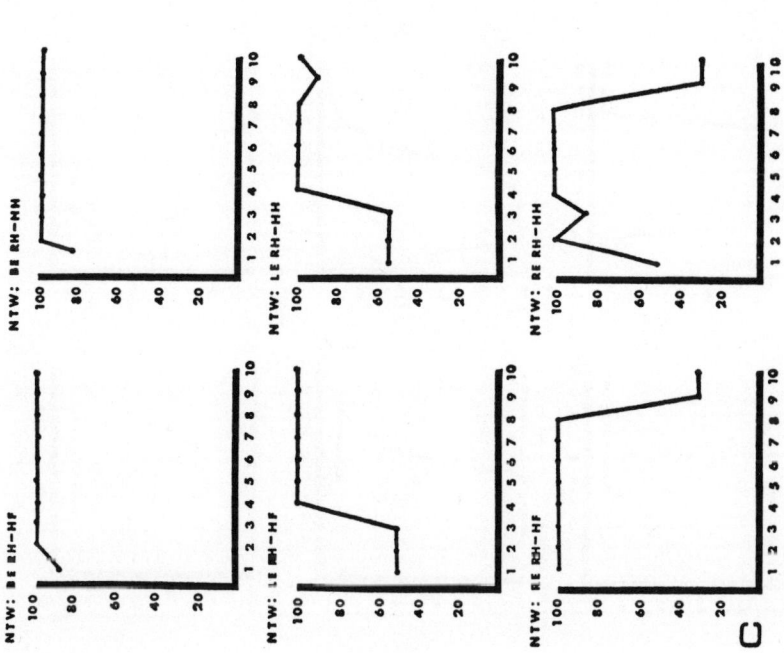

Figure 18. Representative data of control monkeys BNE, CLN, and NTW. The scores indicate percentage correct in approximately ten trials for each lever on the horizontal scale. BE, both eyes open; LE, left eye open; RE, right eye open.

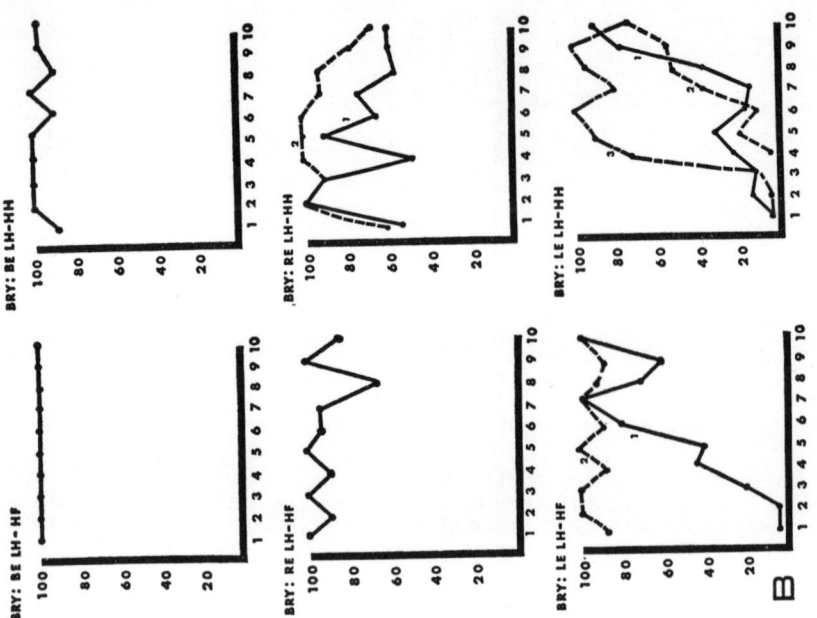

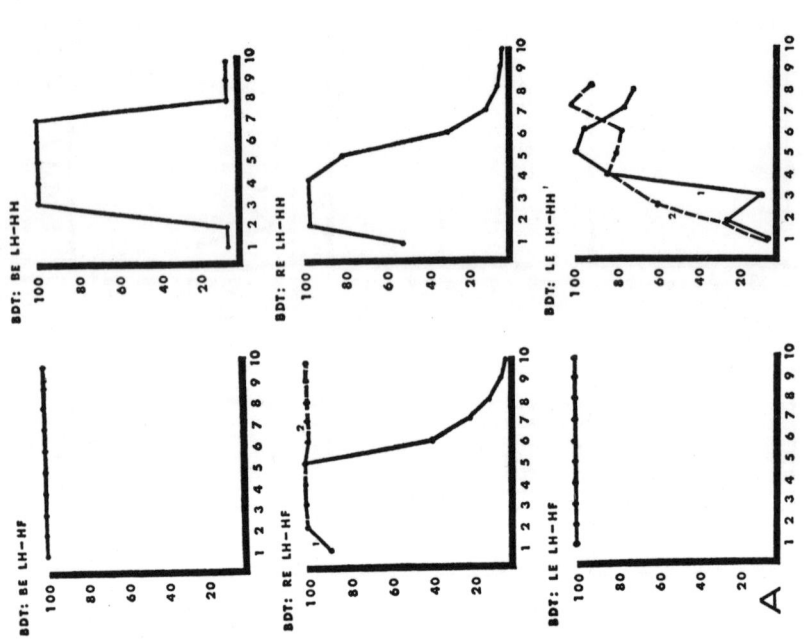

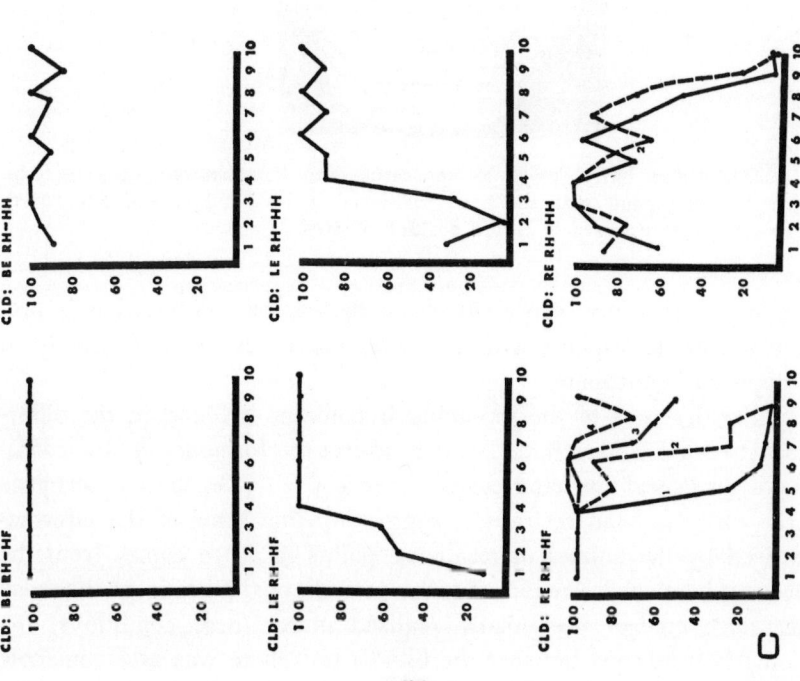

Figure 19. Data on some split-brain monkeys (BDT, BRY, and CLD) with the head either let free (HF) or held (HH) portrayed as in Figure 17. The most erratic and least stable performance is always seen when the head is held in the ipsilateral eye-hand combination. BE, both eyes open; LE, left eye open; RE, right eye open.

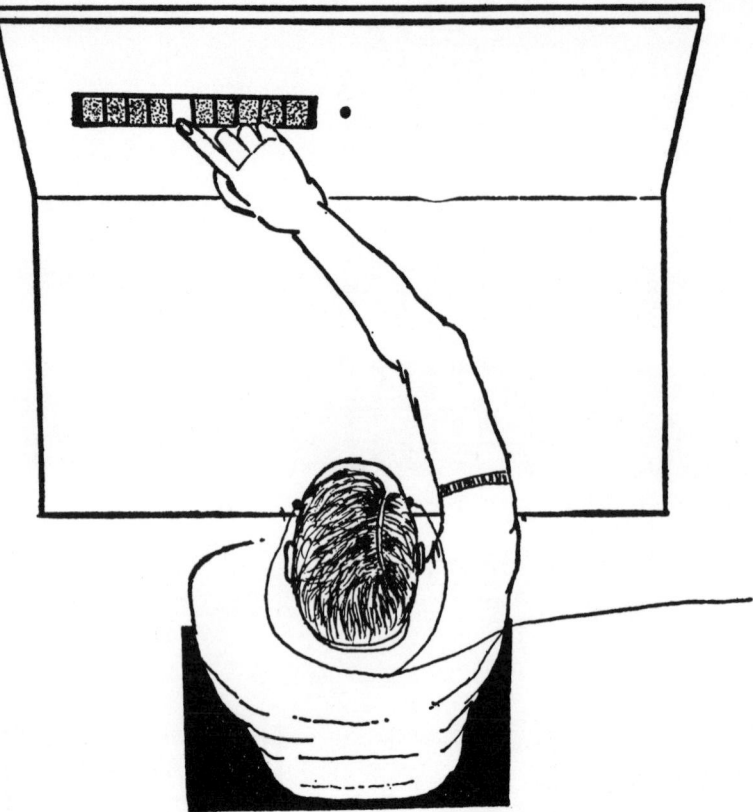

Figure 20. Same basic design as apparatus used in subhuman primate tests. Subject fixates a point with the head positioned in head holder and bite board. Ocular electrodes are used to record position of eyes.

visual-motor response, especially when the sensory information is projected to one hemisphere and the motor control is featured mainly in the opposite hemisphere.

A critical test of the foregoing hypotheses is found in the difference between head-restrained and head-free performance under conditions of ipsilateral eye-hand control. In every case, the animal performs poorly with the head restrained, suggesting that some of the information used by the animal in localizing points in space comes from the nonseeing hemisphere registering the position of the head. At the same time, since control was finally realized under these conditions, the hypothesis would predict that the blind hemisphere was now somehow being cued-in by eye position. Elimination of eye movement in split-brain monkeys would be a difficult procedure. In recent experiments on brain-bisected humans, however, it was shown that eye position contributes dramatically to the overall accuracy of carrying out ipsilateral eye-hand tasks.

The experimental procedure was as follows: Two brain-bisected patients and one normal were studied. The test apparatus is shown in Figure 20. All subjects were positioned in a head holder with a bite board, and were situated 24 inches from the display panel. At the start of each trial, they were instructed to fixate a small light appearing on the vertical meridian. The position of their eyes was monitored, using Beckman ocular electrodes. When fixation was observed to be true and steady, a 100 millisecond light flash was presented on one of ten buttons, falling exclusively into the left visual field.

Two experimental conditions were used. In condition A, the subject with the head fixed was told to look towards the illuminated button and then touch it with the right hand. Under this condition, the stimulus light was *off* before the scan had been made. In condition B, the test was identical, except that the subject was instructed not to look at the illuminated button, but rather to maintain fixation before and during the manual response. In both conditions the light was exclusively flashed to the right hemisphere, but the manual response required the motor system predominately featured in the opposite hemisphere. In the brain-bisected patients, this meant the right hemisphere was attempting to effect control over a motor system that had no direct access to the sensory information.

The results are shown in Figure 21. The normal subject responded easily and well under both conditions, thereby eliminating any possible complications due to procedural artifacts. The brain-bisected patients were accurate in localizing the illuminated point only when eye movements were allowed. When the patients maintained fixation, performance fell to a low level. In addition, the actual hand movements during these latter responses were awkward.

The findings suggest that the final position of the eye is registered in both the left and the right hemispheres. Because the information is available to the left hemisphere, accuracy is possible for right-hand manual responses.

The cross-cuing mechanism proposed appears to be sufficient to explain all previous reports on ipsilateral eye-hand control in cat, monkey, chimpanzee, and man. In all of these preceding studies, save one or two specific tests in man, the theory can account for the behav-

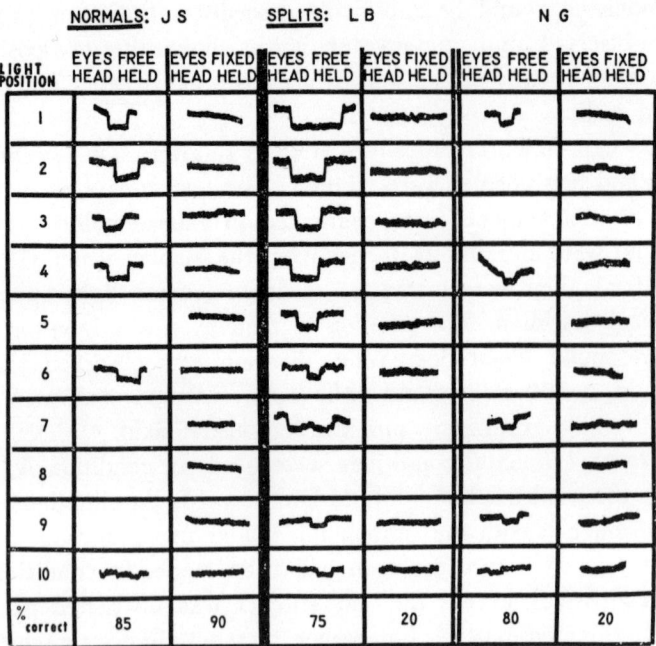

Figure 21. Eye movement recordings of both normal and two split-brain patients. Not all positions were recorded in any 10 trials due to randomizing network generating the stimulus. Percentage of correct scores is based usually on 10 but sometimes 20 trials, with some positions appearing more than once.

ioral data. In the latter case, a specific test as discussed in the foregoing, which required individual responses of the fingers, represents response sequences that cannot be cross-cued.

The implications for these findings in the wider context of the brain mechanisms underlying visual-motor coordination are of interest. It seems abundantly clear that a simple connectionist view of interaction between sensory and motor elements is not helpful in understanding the real circuitry and mechanisms involved. The present data support the earlier view that a general orientation toward a stimulus first takes place involving eye, head, and neck positions, and that this information feeds back and further sets and resets the lower motor apparatus. The view is that sensory-motor integration commences its long sequencing of events in the visual system itself, and that a highly integrated sensory-motor message is delivered to the more clearly efferent motor system controlling specific extremities.

5

Callosal Code

One of the major problems outstanding in split-brain research lies in coming to understand the nature of the callosal code. It is the only fiber tract in the brain that we know transmits high-order information, and any clarification of its processing logic would be of enormous value in attaining clues on the larger question of the brain code. Subsequent to the discovery of the basic phenomena of the split-brain, neuropsychologic studies were carried out with the hope of elucidating the kind, type, and amount of information transmitted by the callosum. More recently, microelectrode analysis of callosal axon response to discrete stimulation of the visual field has been carried out. The basic findings from these areas will be reviewed below. In general, the combined studies do not yet offer much insight into the nature of the problem.

Neuropsychologic Studies

Following the discovery that forebrain commissurotomy blocked the interhemispheric spread of learning and memory, the question remained how chiasm-sectioned but callosum-intact animals performed at a high level following training of one eye-hemisphere and testing of the other. Was a double engram—one formed in each hemisphere— initially layed down, or did one hemisphere learn and the other then "tap" the trained hemisphere during transfer tests?

Most of the experiments run on these and related questions have been carried out in the cat and, as will be seen below, the conclusions reached probably hold only for the cat. In brief, the results suggest that if discriminations are trained to one eye of the chiasm-sectioned cat, subsequent section of the corpus callosum leaves the untrained eye able to perform "simple" tasks, but not more "complex" visual tasks (Myers, 1964). Likewise, subsequent to training a chiasm-sectioned cat simple and complex problems via one eye, lesions in the trained hemisphere leave the other hemisphere able to perform simple, but not complex, discriminations. Additionally, studies inducing conflict by training in opposite valences to similar stimuli seemingly suggest that informational cross talk is of a lower order when taking place between hemispheres through the callosum, but is of a high order within a hemisphere (Myers, 1962). The inference from all these studies has been that the corpus callosum serves as a filter that transmits information but fails on more complex tasks. Therefore, it is concluded that double engrams are laid down for simple discriminations but not for complex tasks. Moreover, since poorer scores are seen in transfer tests with chiasm-sectioned cats on the complex discriminations, it is also concluded that the unilaterally developed engram cannot be tapped as effectively through the callosum.

The foregoing experimental evidence is, in a sense, counterintuitive, especially when considered in the light of the recent split-brain studies on humans. Split visual input into man can be accomplished by having a subject fixate a point. During fixation, all visual information presented to the right of the point is exclusively projected to the left hemisphere and all visual information projected to the left of this point is exclusively projected to the right hemisphere. This being the case, it is difficult, if one views callosal function as presented above, to explain why the normal person is capable of giving a running verbalization of the most complex stimuli falling throughout the entire left visual field. Here, the subject is using the speech center in his left hemisphere to describe complex visual stimulation presented exclusively to the right hemisphere. According to the above experiment, it might be predicted that man could describe only the "simple" aspects of left-field stimulation. Clearly then, it would seem that Myers' experiments on the cat and the inferences from them about the nature of the callosal code do not hold for man.

Surprisingly, no comparable experiments have been carried out using visual tests on the monkey, save for a recent report by Butler (1968). He presents convincing evidence that no difficulties are seen in interocular transfer over a wide range of discriminations. There have been reports that chiasm-sectioned animals do not transfer visual discrimination at a high level (Downer, 1962; Gazzaniga, 1966a; Noble, 1966). But this finding, except in the mirror image experiments of Noble, probably reflects more the nature of the testing situation than the basic underlying neurology and physiology. The experiments that have been run on simple versus complex discriminations have used touch, and in general the finding suggests that the callosum in no way limits simple versus complex discrimination information (Myers, 1964), (However, because of the ipsilateral cuing systems available to the monkey, mentioned in the last chapter, these experiments may not have critically tested the point.)

Some of the issues and problems involved in reconciling the cat and monkey data are as follows. The authors never state in their papers whether or not the complex discrimination was tested first or second during transfer tests. We will assume that the poor performance on the complex discriminations came after the cats were performing well through the untrained eye on the simple discriminations. That is, we will not eliminate the experiment simply on the basis of testing procedure, (i.e., on the possibility that the animal took a few trials to accommodate to the new testing situation).

On the question of double engram formation—one in each hemisphere—the data for the simple discrimination are somewhat convincing. Ablation of the trained hemisphere leaves the untrained eye able to perform at a high level. At the same time, the transfer tests in the "train, cut callosum, test untrained eye" experiment are less compelling. Of the four cats used, three had prior experience with the problem using the untrained eye. In addition, transfer scores on two of the four cats were somewhat equivocal.

The inability to demonstrate double engram formation with complex tests is shaky. The original data are sparse, but do suggest that testing through the untrained eye yields poorer performance when compared to the simple task. Whether this reflects a property of the hemispheric communication system per se remains obscure. It may well be that the results point up the type of visual deficits produced in the cat following chiasm sectioning. Stone (1966) in studies on the cat has demonstrated that a chiasm sectioning would severly limit the visual input to each hemisphere, to a degree that surpasses the deficit produced by similar surgery in monkey and man. Not only do 100 percent of the nasal fibers cross in the chiasm, but also approximately 25 percent of the temporal fibers.

When this is taken into account, along with the neurophysiologic observations on recordings in the splenium, reported below, which show that responses are found only in the midline of the visual field, the inference made from the behavioral findings becomes tenuous indeed. Clearly, it could be maintained that the chiasm section simultaneously reduces overall visual input, and as a result greatly impairs the efficiency of the intact callosum.

Taken as a whole, the general impression that the callosum has severe limits on its informational capacity simply does not hold for monkey and man, and the results on the cat are somewhat debatable. Likewise, whether or not double or single engrams are laid down during pre-commissure-section training seems also to be an open question. Certainly, some engrams are singly laid down, such as speech and language; and some evidence exists that visual discriminations in the normal monkeys are laid down unilaterally (Gazzaniga, 1963).

Another approach used in the analysis of callosal function has been to define and localize which areas are critically involved in the transfer of visual and tactual training. Experimentally, observations have been made on the cat and monkey. There is also some clinical evidence available in the literature which comments on the question. The general view is that the interhemispheric transfer of visual pattern learning is abolished by section of the middle two-thirds of the callosum. The function of the anterior half of the callosum has remained a mystery.

The experimental results in this area of research are not without their problems. Usually, animals were used and they underwent surgical disconnection of a part of the callosum. They were subsequently trained on a visual or a tactual discrimination in one hemisphere, tested through the other hemisphere, and then sacrificed. While this approach admittedly answers the question of the effects of partial commissure section on the transfer of one (and sometimes two) visual or tactual discrimination, it leaves wide open the question of how more experienced animals would perform. It is clear from a variety of both formal and informal observations that split-brain animals simply change their strategies and adopt new modes of coping with problems as their overall experience in training progresses. With this in mind, it becomes difficult to interpret whether the effects of partial callosal sectioning reflect an interruption of a basic neurologic process or reflect a disruption of a particular psychologic strategy apparent at the time of testing.

Another complication in this kind of analysis of callosal function lies in teasing out the contributions of the callosum versus some of the other forebrain commissures. In particular, this becomes extremely difficult when trying to ascribe specific functions to various areas of the callosum overlying the hippocampal commissure. When this part of the callosum is cut, the hippocampal commissure is almost invariably sectioned. When deficits are observed subsequent to this kind of surgery it is, of course, unclear whether it was a callosal or hippocampal commissure lesion that produced the particular syndrome observed. Some suggestions do exist in my own unpublished data that the hippocampus may be critically involved in the interhemispheric transfer of visual learning. Certainly it is a structure that is extremely important in the learning process, and its commissural connections must be transmitting some kind of information that is usable to the untrained halfbrain. Determining the relationships between these two commissures would be a fascinating problem and one of many that remain to be done.

In general, partial callosum-sectioning studies indicate that visual discriminations are not transferred if the posterior portion of the callosum is sectioned. In the cat, 6.2 mm or 44 percent (moving anteriorly from the splenium) of the callosum must be sectioned before transfer is stopped. This correlates favorably with the anatomy of the cat, thus indicating that lesions in the occipital lobe produce heavy degeneration in the splenium and then continue in diminishing amounts up to the middle of the splenium. Curiously, sectioning of the anterior portion all the way back, including 87 percent of the callosum, also prevents transfer of visual discriminations in the cat according to Myers (1962), even though a good deal of the splenium is left intact. Whether this view will hold up is another question, for the data on both of these points come from two animals. With this level of confidence understood, it could be guessed that in the cat the splenium is not involved at all—having been eliminated for purposes of transfer by the chiasm section, with the resulting loss of foveal fibers. It is conceivable that a 2 to 3 mm section floating slightly anterior to the posterior tip might eliminate transfer in the cat.

Unfortunately, the foregoing analysis does not strictly hold for

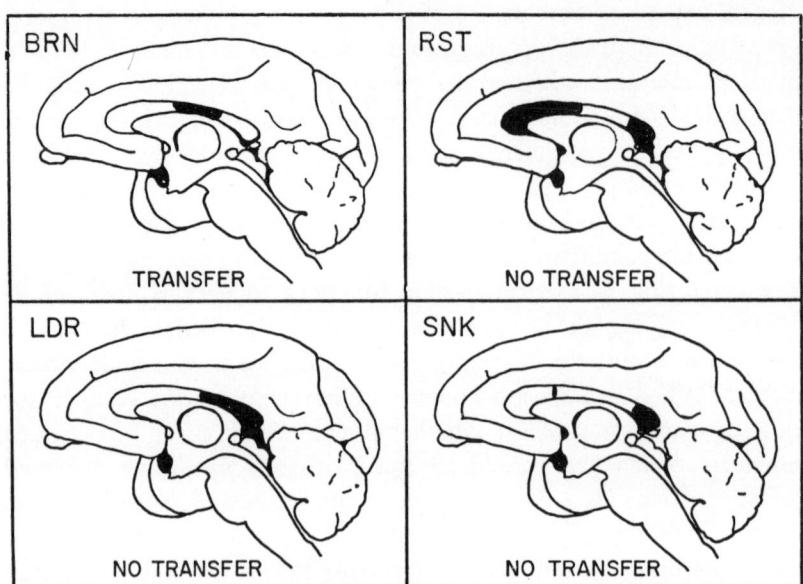

Figure 22. Sagittal sections of monkey brains, showing extended neocortical commissure surgery needed to block interhemispheric transfer of visual learning using positive reinforcement. In animal SNK, section of the splenium alone stopped transfer only temporarily. Permanent blockage was possible when the anterior commissure was also sectioned.

the monkey. In the experiments most closely related in design to those in the cat, just the splenium and the anterior commissure of the chimpanzee were found to be critically involved in transfer of pattern discriminations (Black and Myers, 1964). In another series of experiments in monkeys (where animals were trained on several discriminations) this observation was confirmed and extended, in that it was observed that a partial section of the callosum (Fig. 22) temporarily abolished transfer (Gazzaniga, 1966a). After the first discrimination, however, transfer again appeared. Subsequent sectioning of the anterior commissure appeared to completely eliminate pattern-discrimination transfer. The data are consistent with a notion that one is working with an ever changing system, and that when one avenue of interhemispheric communication is blocked up, the animal adapts a different neurologic, if not psychologic, strategy, and proceeds, using other available mechanisms.

In addition to the above, the data from primates suggest that if any portion of the splenium is left intact, regardless of how much of the anterior portion of the callosum is sectioned, interhemispheric transfer will readily occur on visual discriminations.

Surveys of the clinical literature by Bremer et al. (1956) and more recently by Geschwind (1965 a, b) have been extremely fruitful. Both have pointed up Maspes' (1948) observation that section of the splenium in man results in the left hemisphere being unable to read words and letters presented in the left visual field (right hemisphere). Yet these same patients could describe colors, objects, and other visual stimuli presented in the same visual field. Trescher and Ford (1937) had earlier described a case that showed similar disturbances. These basic observations have been observed in a most dramatic, fascinating report by Professor James G. Taylor. In a self diagnosis made in a letter to me, he recalled an experience he had as a young boy.

> . . . I am reminded of a curious kind of "hemianopsia" that I occasionally suffered in my youth—probably some form of migrane. I was scarcely aware of any visual disturbance until I tried to read. The printed symbols to the right of the fixation point had vanished, and I made wild guesses as to the identity of unseen or partly seen words, just as your subjects did. The order is the reverse of what you found, but it is probably that my speech centre is in the right hemisphere, since the right side of my body is deformed, and has been weaker than the left from infancy. My difficulty in reading could have been due to a temporary blocking of commissural transmission from left to right. . . . Though the events occurred more than 50 years ago, the experience was so striking that I have retained a vivid memory of it. The first attack occurred when I was a high-school student. I was aware of nothing until the English master asked me to read something aloud. Normally I could read quite fluently, but on this occasion I stumbled so badly and uttered so many words that were not in the text that the master terminated the exercise in a hurry. My memory is very distinct on the point that the difficulty was not due to a blurring of the print. It was a form of amblyopia. There was just a total absence of print to the right of the fixation point, and not even a darkening of the page to indicate that there was something there. It was as if my left eye shut, and the right blind spot had increased in area until it reached the boundary of the fovea.

In other words, the experience was exactly like the disappearance of a small object in the blind spot. Of course, I knew that there must be printed matter there, but it remained invisible until the next saccade translated it to the left visual field.

It has been suggested that the reason why Maspes' patient could verbally describe colors and objects but not letters and words lies in the fact that the right hemisphere cannot elaborate the visual-verbal material, whereas it can elaborate and make rich associations for objects. In the former case, the raw visual stimulus can neither get over to the left hemisphere for interpretation through traditionally visual pathways because of the splenium section, nor can it be elaborated in the right hemisphere, because of that hemisphere's lack of the proper verbal machinery. The objects can be described, however, because the right hemisphere can elaborate that kind of visual stimulus, and subsequent to this processing can send the critical information about it to the left hemisphere through more anterior (and uncut) portions of the callosum. This is an intriguing suggestion, and a parallel can be drawn between this kind of interpretation of the human data and some recent studies on the monkey. Studies by Hamilton et al. (1968) and Sperry and Green (1966) have indicated that callosal segments anterior to the splenium, when left intact, allow split-brain monkeys to make visual-visual comparisons. Yet, these same monkeys, when tested for a transfer of a particular discrimination from one hemisphere to the other, performed poorly. In other experiments, where it was shown that spilt-brain monkeys can process more information in a given instant of time than normals, it was observed that an animal with the splenium intact performed just as well as a total split (Gazzaniga and Young, 1967). In one sense, these studies suggest that the more integrated or associative a particular perceptual task is, the more important the anterior portions of the callosum become.

Transfer With Shock Avoidance

In a series of experiments carried out using shock avoidance, it has been reported that visual pattern discrimination does transfer at a high level in the cat (Sechzer, 1964). That is, when negative reinforcement is in order instead of the positive reward paradigm generally used, enormous savings are observed when the untrained hemisphere is tested for transfer. While these results are extremely interesting they are not to be accepted without caution, for clear differences in the nature of the preparations exist. For example, not all the cats used in this study had the anterior commissure sectioned! The distinct possibility remains that transfer would be impaired if the anterior commissure had been included in the original surgery. It should be recalled that leaving the anterior commissure intact in the monkey results in savings when using positive food reward.

Recently Doty (1969) has made related observations in the monkey. Using the techniques of intercranial conditioning, monkeys failed to transfer using positive reinforcement when the corpus callosum was sectioned but the anterior commissure was left intact. Using shock avoidance, transfer was seen but was subsequently abolished when the anterior commissure was sectioned.

It remains an open question, of course, whether the transfer obtained with shock avoidance reflects transfer of information per se across the anterior commissure. The training technique might well simply serve to alert the untrained hemisphere to pay "rapt attention" to an upcoming cue and to learn its significance quickly. One-trial learning is commonly seen in the cat and monkey in the open field under more natural life circumstances. Perhaps shock avoidance provides a similar state of affairs for the animal in the laboratory.

Neurophysiologic Studies

Microelectrode analysis of callosal neurons has revealed several interesting characteristics of the system (Berlucchi et al., 1967; Hubel and Wiesel, 1967). To date, studies have examined only the visual interhemispheric connections in the cat. To be sure, there have been a host of other electrophysiologic experiments on the callosum, but most of these, as presently understood, do not bear directly on the issues raised by the neuropsychologic experiments.

Single cell recordings in the splenium have revealed the following (Fig. 23): simple, complex, and hypercomplex type units, reminiscent of the kind observed by Hubel and Wiesel (1962) were found in the splenium, but not in the more anterior portions of the callosum. All responses recorded were on or about the midline of the visual field—and observation in basic agreement with that of Whitteridge (1965)

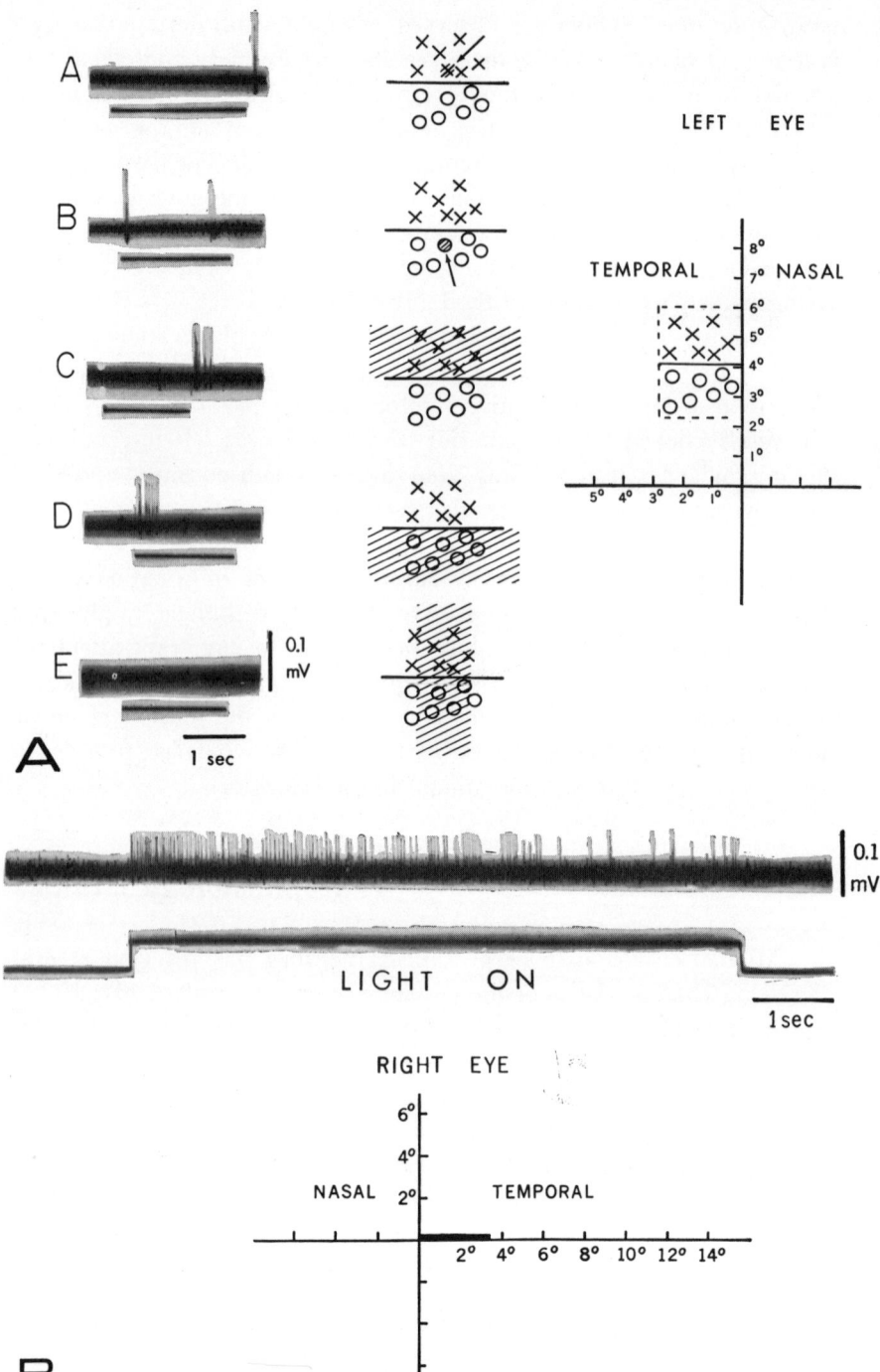

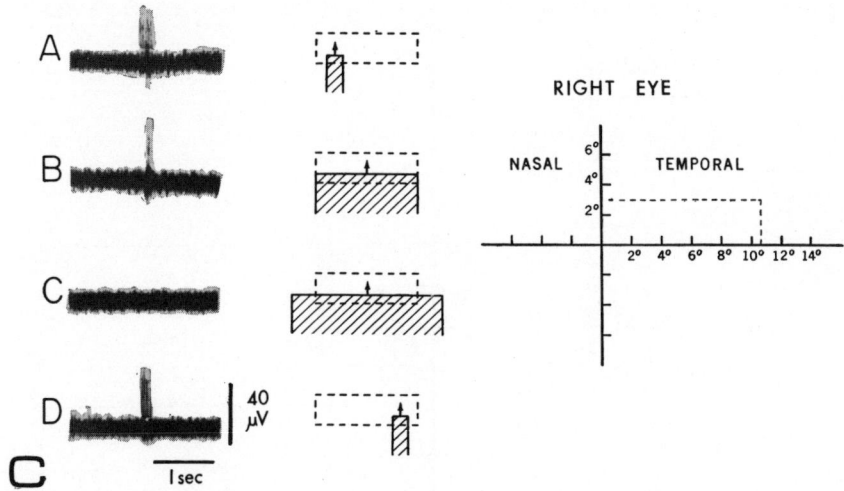

Figure 23. A. Example of callosal unit having a simple visual receptive field: this unit was driven from the left eye only. The receptive field (shown at the right of the figure) was divided by a straight line in an upper excitatory region and a lower inhibitory region. A and B show off- and on-responses to small (42′) spots of light shone in the positions indicated by the arrows in the drawings at the right of the records. Similar on- and off-responses were recorded upon illumination of other points marked with circles and crosses respectively. C and D show increased off- and on-responses to stimuli covering the entire excitatory and inhibitory areas respectively (spike amplitude is reduced compared to A and B because the records were taken several minutes after the latter). E shows absence of response to simultaneous illumination of both antagonistic areas of the receptive field. B. Example of callosal unit having a complex visual receptive field: this unit was driven from right eye only. It did not respond to spots of light shone in the receptive field (shown at bottom of figure). The optimal stimulus was a horizontal edge (light up) shone in the receptive field. The length of this edge could be prolonged beyond the vertical boundaries of the receptive field with full preservation of the response. C. Example of callosal unit having a hypercomplex receptive field: this unit was driven from the right eye. The best stimulus was a narrow (1° 45′) band of light moved vertically upward anywhere in the receptive field (shown at right of figure): A and D. Increasing field led to a decrease of the response (B): absence of response was observed upon extension of the width of the stimulus beyond the boundaries of the receptive field (C). (From Berlucci et al. 1967. *Arch. Ital. Biol.*, 105:583-596.)

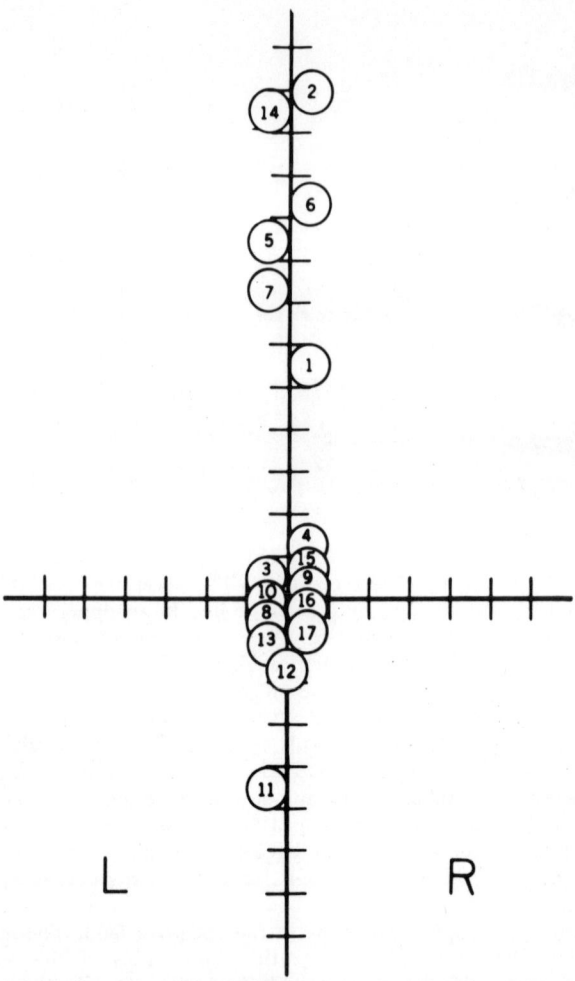

Figure 24. Relation of receptive fields of callosal units to the vertical meridian of the visual field. Each circle indicates the position of the receptive field of the corresponding callosal unit (indicated by number) in the visual field, independently of its shape and size. In case of large receptive fields, the circle shows only the position of that part of the field located in close contact with the vertical meridian. Apparent absence of callosal receptive fields in the lower portion of the visual field is due to obstruction of vision of this area by the head holder. The position of fields in area centralis is highly schematized; in fact, most fields in this area showed an almost total overlapping. Each division on the coordinates corresponds to 2°. (From Berlucci et al. 1967. *Arch. Ital. Biol.*, 538-596.)

(Fig. 24). In a more recent study on chiasm-sectioned cats, Berlucchi and Rizzoletti (1968) demonstrated that units recorded in visual cortex, and responding to midline stimulation, received an input via the callosum. Covering one eye during testing would find a particular unit responding only to information present in its ipsilateral field, and no responses were evident across the midline.

These findings raise interesting questions about the nature of the callosal code. Does the callosum merely serve to unite the two visual fields in the midline? Put differently, is the midline the only aspect of the external world regarding which the callosum can communicate interhemispherically? These interpretations seem difficult to conceptualize. As we can easily attest, visual information to the left of fixation and quite far away from the visual midline can be described through speech, which usually depends on the left hemisphere. In one sense, the question becomes: Is the left hemisphere simultaneously aware of the information presented to the right hemisphere, because a duplicate picture is sent over via the callosum? Or is it that the right hemisphere alone is aware of the left field, and that a spoken description (coming from the left hemisphere) of what was presented to the right is possible only because the right hemisphere continually sends over a running description of what is happening in some kind of abstract form, and in some kind of code? The simple analogy to the latter hypothesis would be the situation where two people are looking at different aspects of a scene. Each is directly aware of his own visual sphere, but is aware of his neighbor's only to the extent that he listens to a description of it. While there simply are not enough data to distinguish between these different interpretations of the phenomenon, there are certain appealing aspects to this latter interpretation. It would seem redundant that the brain should send a duplicate picture of the visual information to the other hemisphere, when it is primarily projected to the one.

An observation related to the above is the peculiar phenomenon that split-brain patients do not complain about their inability to verbally describe visual information to the left of fixation. Imagine yourself the day before undergoing split-brain surgery looking about the hospital room with all the perceptional unity imaginable. When looking at a person's face you not only see everything to the right of fixation, which goes to the left hemisphere, but also, of course, his left half face. After surgery, everything you would find much the same except that your left speech hemisphere would now be unable to describe the part of the person's face falling to the left of fixation. With intact half-brains like ours, it seems incomprehensible that we would not notice a difference in our visual world. Yet, split, the left hemisphere never complains, never alludes to a difficulty. It is as if the mechanism for the realization that vision was once available across the midline exists only when the callosum is intact. With it gone, the left hemisphere simply doesn't respond to an appropriate question about this subject from the examiner. Indeed, one would miss the departure of a good friend more, apparently, than the left hemisphere misses the right.

SUMMARY

By way of summary of the foregoing, a few questions will be considered. Does the callosal-intact cat, monkey, or man lay down bilateral engrams when training has been limited to one hemisphere? The evidence would suggest that it does not always do so. In the cat, there is some evidence for this view. In the monkey, the only available data suggest that visual discriminations learned preoperatively can be performed by only one hemisphere postoperatively. (It is most likely that this is a threshold phenomenon, probably dependent on such variables as the nature of the stimulus, the amount of overtraining, and the type of reinforcement used during initial training.) There is some evidence that tactile discriminations are layed down bilaterally in the monkey. In man, both single and double engram formation are apparent.

Is there a limit or load capacity on the kinds and types of information that can be transmitted to the callosum? The original observations were made on the cat and in retrospect, there are some reasons to question the overall impression of information limitation. There is little or no evidence that this is the case in monkey, and in man it clearly is not the case.

Lastly, is there evidence that the callosum transmits in some kind of spatial-temporal code the "stuff" of learning? Put differently, does the callosum induce the learning and memory, trained to one hemisphere, into the other? On this point, there is no concrete evidence. The most parsimonious explanation would be that no such phenomenon is apparent. Rather, when the chiasm-sectioned, callosum-intact animal lays down bilateral engrams, each hemisphere during the original training period, works in concert. Each uses the raw stimulus information, with the untrained hemisphere receiving its information in some kind of abstract code through the corpus callosum.

In any real sense, the question that we have asked ourselves is no smaller than the general question of the nature of the brain code. The logic of information transmission and storage in the nervous system will certainly be a step closer to being understood when the properties of forebrain commissures are more clearly elucidated. At present these properties are as mysterious today as ever before.

6

Psychologic and Neurologic Effects of Cerebral Bisection in Man

Past reports concerning the effects of lesions in the human corpus calsum have been inconsistent. Observations pointing to the presence of a distinct functional syndrome of the corpus callosum in patients with vascular or neoplastic lesions or with surgical section of the corpus callosum (Geschwind and Kaplan, 1962) have been largely outweighed by more extensive studies in which no apraxia, agnosia, agraphia, or other mental syndromes could be observed after surgical section of the corpus callosum (Akelaitis, 1941, 1943, 1944; Akelaitis et al., 1942; Bridgeman and Smith, 1945). From the numerous animal studies, however, it has become clear that the corpus callosum in cats, monkeys, and chimpanzees plays a definite and important role in the cross-integration of a variety of sensory, motor, and associated functions involving interaction between the two hemispheres.

In this chapter, the body of evidence collected from the recent series of studies on callosum-sectioned patients will be reviewed and up-dated, using the general format put forth in the original reports. In particular, those areas involving language, information process analysis, as well as more basic observations on somatosensory function, will be extensively expanded over the original reports (Gazzaniga et al., 1962, 1963, 1965, 1967; Gazzaniga and Sperry, 1967). The neurologic findings will be followed by the psychological observations made on each separated hemisphere.

Case Histories

All the patients in the present series underwent surgery in an effort to control epileptic seizures. The idea was that seizure activity commencing in one hemisphere could be localized and contained, thereby leaving the other hemisphere seizure free, and able to maintain basic, normative bodily functions. Early reports on the therapeutic advantages of callosal surgery are confused (Akelaitis, 1941). Careful analysis of the published reports carried out by Bogen (1960, personal communication) revealed that as much evidence existed for beneficial effects as did against such effects. In addition, only one case of the 26 reported by Akelaitis had both the corpus callosum and anterior commissure sectioned, thereby leaving open a greater number of avenues for the interhemispheric spread of seizures. All of the present series of cases had both the corpus callosum and the anterior commissure sectioned.

Case W. J. was the first patient. After extensive medical and neurologic testing, which lasted for approximately two years prior to surgery and included trips to the National Institutes of Health for special tests, it was finally concluded that all other opportunities for permanently abolishing the seizures appeared closed. Subsequently, each case was given similar thorough workups before the final decision to operate was made.

In all, ten cases have undergone midline sectioning of the corpus callosum and anterior commissure. Data on three of the ten will be presented in the following discussion. Three others were frequently tested, and all showed the main features of the disconnection syndrome. However, as the testing procedures became more sophisticated and time consuming, only the cases with more or less pure commissural lesions as well as a smooth and quick postoperative recovery course were examined thoroughly. The remaining four cases experienced postoperative complications that mainly reflected physiologic conditions not associated with the craniotomy. Extensive medical descriptions of the patients have been published elsewhere (Bogen and Vogel, 1962, 1963; Bogen, Fisher, and Vogel, 1965).

CASE I:

The patient, a 48-year-old male war veteran, had been having grand mal convulsions for ten years subsequent to injuries received in 1944. His first blackout spells occurred shortly after a parachute jump over Germany during a bombing raid. Incomplete opening of the parachute resulted in several fractures of the left leg and unconsciousness of unknown duration. During subsequent internment in a German camp, he was rendered unconscious by a rifle blow to the left parietal region and during this time he suffered from malnutrition, losing nearly 80 pounds. He developed dystrophic skin changes in both hands along with widespread, moderate muscle atrophy.

The seizures were refractory to medical management, with a frequency of at best about one per week and at worst about seven to ten per day, culminating in status epilepticus every two to three months. The onset of seizures was often clearly related to emotional upset, and a hysterical element has sometimes been inferred from the bizarre pattern. Electroencephalograms have often shown a left temporal-parietal focus as well as consistent bitemporal abnormality.

He was right-handed, had an I.Q. of 113, and in both pre- and postoperative testing, the patient revealed a high intellectual level plus a good sense of humor, and a keen interest in his surroundings. He was relatively well read, his favorite author being Victor Hugo, and he kept apace of current events, showing special interest in the moon shot.

With regard to somesthesis, it was shown in preoperative testing that the patient when blindfolded could describe or correctly name various objects, such as coins and kitchen utensils, held in either hand, and with either hand could write the name of the object held in the opposite hand. Occasional errors were recorded in the discrimination between similar sized coins with the left hand, e.g., between a dime and a penny.

Visual testing before the operation showed that the patient had uncorrected acuity of 20/70 O.D. plus 10.v., and 20/50 O.S.[1] Exten-

---

[1] The optometric tests were performed by Dr. G. Kambara.

sive tests, including perimetry, showed no abnormality except some jerkiness of motion. Tachistoscopic presentations of letters, numbers, geometric figures, and sentences showed that all stimuli were easily recognized and interpreted correctly in either half-field and/or correctly recorded by manual response with either hand. His reading in general was normal.

Motor responses of all kinds to verbal commands were carried out accurately and with no gross impairments observed in either hand. He could, for example, write dictation moderately well with the left hand as well as the right.

At the time of the operation in February of 1961, extracallosal damage, which included atrophy of the right frontal lobe, was judged by the surgeons to be present. There also may have been damage to the right fornix. The corpus callosum, anterior commissure, and hippocampal commissure were sectioned. Immediately after surgery, generalized weakness, akinesis, and mutism were evident, but had largely disappeared when postoperative testing was started one month after surgery. Anticonvulsive medication was reinstated shortly after surgery. There have since been several brief attacks with loss of consciousness, but as yet no major convulsions. Occasional brief episodes of clonic-like tremors confined to the distal portions of the right arm or leg have also been noted postoperatively. The operation appears to have left no gross changes in temperament or intellect and the patient has repeatedly remarked that he feels better, generally, than he has in years.

CASE II:

The patient, a 30-year-old housewife, has two children and a concerned and intelligent husband. Her convulsions were first observed in 1951 when she was 18 years old, shortly after her marriage. Her grandmother is recorded to have had severe epileptic seizures, and her daughter is now being treated for seizures. For seven or so years after their first observance the convulsions occurred usually at a frequency of one per month, and were correlated with the onset of the patient's menstrual period. They occurred usually in the evening and they were severe in nature, causing the patient to be bedridden for two to three days afterwards. In the early 1960's the complexion of her convulsions changed. She would have intermittent convulsions for an entire week at a time and would have to be admitted to the hospital for extensive medication. This sort of seizure pattern persisted until immediately prior to the operation.

She scored with an I.Q. of 74 and always displayed a good, friendly nature along with a definite slapstick sort of humor. She had a very low motivational level, and failing to complete a simple task, she would usually give up. The registered I.Q. of 74, however, was not felt to be a good evaluation of her general intelligence. Subsequent administration of various aspects of the test revealed that she was capable of quite higher scores in certain parts, if the instructions were made absolutely clear to the patient before starting a particular task. However, there is no question that the patient was a relatively dull and submissive sort, with little regard for the subtle aspects of human activities.

Preoperative testing with regard to somesthesis showed that the patient had a mild hypoesthesia on the left side. She was completely able, however, to identify objects held in each hand and to cross-localize points of stimulation over the entire body. Pain and temperature discriminations were also carried out equally well on both sides of the body. Visual testing revealed a normal perimetry. There were no motor problems, and all actions to verbal commands were easily carried out by both arms and both legs.

At the time of the operation, the entire corpus callosum and anterior commissure were sectioned along with the massa intermedia. The right fornix was also cut. There was no atrophy apparent at the time of the operation; areas of calcification, however, were seen in x-rays in the right hemisphere. The patient's postoperative recovery was good. Within a week, she was up, walking around the hospital and eating without any help. However, for up to two weeks after the operation, the patient displayed labile affect. At one moment, for example, she would be explaining some previous experience and would talk in a normal manner. Suddenly she would be on the verge of tears, all the while keeping the main train of thought of the conversation. Then, just as abruptly, she would resume talking in a normal fashion.

During this period, she was prone to much confabulation. When asked, for example, who Dr. Vogel was, she replied, "A brain doctor." When asked if he had been to see her, she replied, "Yes, in fact he took me to the store." When she was challenged on this, she kept maintaining that she had been taken to the market by Dr. Vogel. She then said (to her mother, who was also present), that she felt she had been drinking too much. She seemed to have a good memory and after the operation easily picked me out from a group of people when we entered the room. She also appeared to have good postoperative memory for

PSYCHOLOGIC AND NEUROLOGIC EFFECTS 79

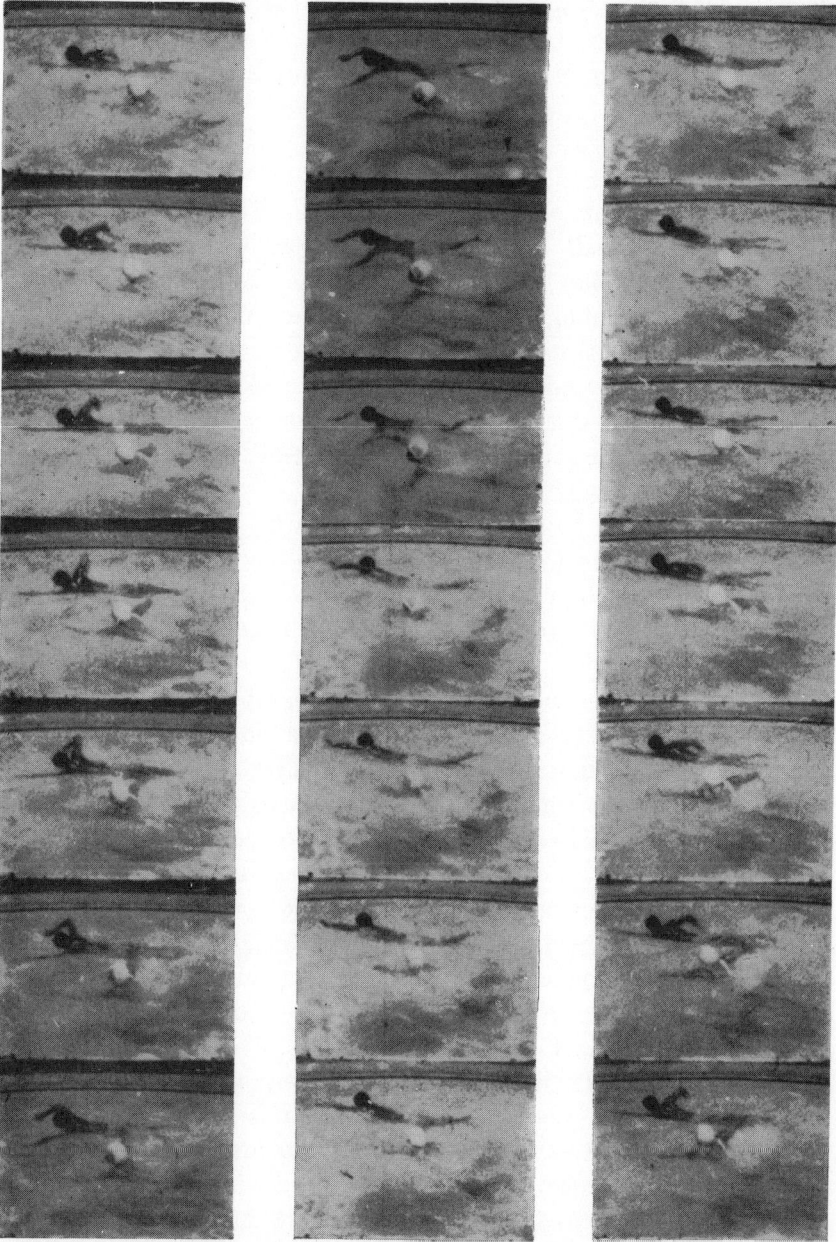

Figure 25. Which one has the split? Husband and wife swimming. The wife is Case II about 8 months after surgery. She has little problem keeping up with her husband in a free-style swim race.

much of her past, and was able to hum several of her old favorite songs, such as "Sleepy Lagoon." Her retention of motor coordination, eight months after surgery, is demonstrated in Figure 25.

CASE III:

The patient, an obviously very bright, affable, happy, and for the most part normally developed boy, was 12 years old at the time of surgery. His hobbies include drawing, swimming, and other physical activities such as skating and some other games. At the time of surgery, he attended public school and was in the seventh grade. He had no problem in reading, and quite readily read a passage full of terms not ordinarily read by a boy of his age. His pronunciation was good, but he seemed to have a general speech impediment, which appeared as a slight slur when saying some words.

Preoperatively, he drew Necker cubes with either hand. He was right-handed, could write with his right hand, and to a lesser degree with his left. He delighted in making sketches, and aspired some day to be a cartoonist. There was some doubt whether the limited artistic ability he possessed was not more contrived than real.

The patient had no problem identifying objects in either hand. He had no problem cross-localizing from one side of the body to the other. There were indications of a slight general hypoesthesia. When words were flashed in either visual field, he read them off with ease.

According to his parents, his seizures started at the age of three years. His severe seizures began about six months before surgery. He was placed on heavier medication, but this did not seem to help. However, he was so drugged by the increased dosage, that he would fall to sleep frequently in class. Under lighter dosage, his parents claimed he was a talkative, active child at home. They also claimed that he had certain psychologic difficulties with his playmates. They claimed he didn't do very well in school, with C being the average grade; he frequently had lower grades. There was no question that he was capable of far better grades, for he scored 115 on the Wechsler Intelligence Scale for Children. He, in fact, maintained that he was simply lazy and chose not to work for the higher grade. He claimed some of the children didn't like him and didn't want to be bothered with him. He said, "When they feel that way, I feel that way towards them." He reports all of this in a cheerful mood. The surgeon's notes indicate an uncomplicated operation. No major veins were ligated and there was no serious bleeding.

On the first postoperative day, the patient woke up and asked if he had had an EEG the preceding day. The doctor said no, he had had surgery. He said, "Oh, that explains my splitting headache." His speech was not only fluent but of the same type and aptitude that he possessed preoperatively. For example, he was able to say rapidly, "Peter Piper picked a peck of pickled peppers; a peck of pickled peppers Peter Piper picked." He appeared to be his same humorous self. He complained about the catheter: "It is not very pleasant to have something stuck up your penis." His ability to control the left side of his body was extremely good. He could hold up his left hand and he had a grasp reflex on both sides. However, when asked to hold up two fingers with his left hand he failed. He recognized touch on only the right side of the body, not the left. The patient was talkative and normally complaining about the general condition a patient finds himself in after a craniotomy. It could almost be said that if the patient did not have a bandage on his head, he (as revealed through his speech and general behavior), would be indistinguishable from his preoperative self.

Neurologic Findings

OBSERVATIONS OF SOMESTHESIS

Considerable uncertainty exists regarding the nature of somatosensory representation in the cerebral cortex of primates and other mammals, particularly with respect to the presence and significance of ipsilateral components. There is general agreement to the extent that cerebral projection of the various somatic afferent systems is largely contralateral for all regions of the body, excepting the neck and head, which are bilaterally represented through the ascending pathways of nerve V.

Evidence regarding the presence and extent of ipsilateral representation for the trunk and limbs is less consistent. Survival of at least crude sensitivity to stimuli after hemispherectomy on the affected side in the cat and monkey suggests the presence of significant ipsilateral representation. Survival of somatosensory functions is likely to be particularly good following hemispherectomies for infantile hemiplegia, suggesting that potential ipsilateral pathways may lie dormant or underdeveloped in the normal brain (White et al., 1959; Gardner et al., 1955). Studies of humans with penetrating brain wounds have suggested a more diffuse and bilateral representation for the left hand than for the right (Semmes et al., 1960). The presence of some ipsilateral projection is supported also from both anatomic and electrophysiologic studies, particularly with reference to the spinothalamic system now believed to contain some touch and pressure components (Rose and Mountcastle, 1960).

The following observations provide further evidence bearing on these and related questions: somatosensory tests were administered that relate to the laterality of cortical representation and the cross-integration of somesthetic information from one to the other side of the body. In general, the results demonstrate the importance of the corpus callosum for such cross-integration, but also give information concerning the type and amount of ipsilateral representation present following brain bisection. Additionally, these studies would suggest that the presence and extent of the ipsilateral component appear to vary and change during the postoperative course—with greater capacities being observed in the second and third postoperative years. This is not to suggest that a fundamental change is occurring in the underlying neurologic mechanism. Rather, it appears to reflect in part the increasing awareness that patients pay to a variety of psychologic strategies available to them, allowing them to get more out of what ipsilateral representation they normally possess.

Localization of Light Touch

With vision eliminated by a blindfold, the subjects were required to localize, by pointing with their finger, the spot on the skin at which a brief, light, tactile stimulus was applied. In most of the tests, the patients were verbally instructed to use either the right hand or the left hand as designated by the experimenter. In other tests, free use of either hand was allowed, and in others, verbal reports of the stimulus locus were obtained.

Throughout all phases of testing, the patients were able to find points of stimulation if both the stimulus and the response were kept to the same side of the body. If the patients were responding with the left hand, for example, all points of stimulation on their left foot, leg, trunk, arm, hand, and face were found with reasonable accuracy. They could locate accurately, with the left thumb, points of stimulation among the left fingers, and did so by responding immediately and also with a 5-, 10-, or 20-second delay imposed.

With no restrictions placed on hand use, the patients generally used the left hand for any point on the left half of the body and the right hand for any point on the right side, except in the facial region, where either hand was used with seeming equal facility. Correct spoken description of the locus of stimulation was consistently observed for points on the right extremities, right-half trunk, and the head. Cases II and III were also able almost from the beginning to describe stimulation points over the entire left-half body, except for the hand and foot. Good spoken accounts of left-sided stimulation for Case I, however, were not possible.

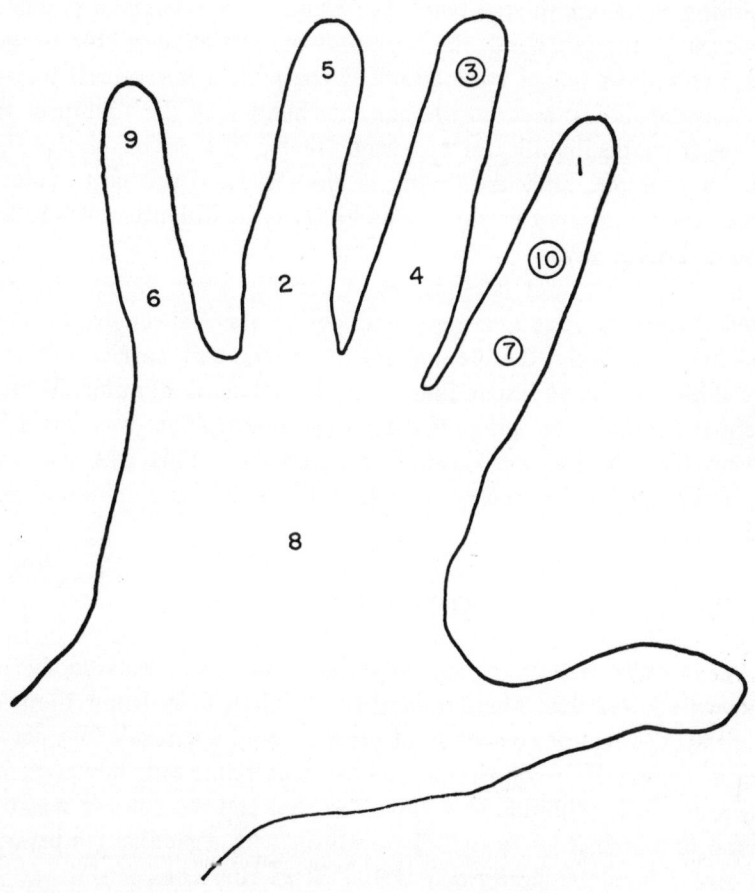

Figure 26. Figure shows points of stimulation on palmar surface of hand A. Hand B, using its thumb, was to find the corresponding point. Only those points circled were correct on this particular test sequence.

In early cross-localization testing, all patients performed poorly. With the left hand, the patients were unable to localize points on the right foot, leg, arm, hand, and the half of the trunk. In many instances, when the right leg or hand was stimulated, the patients failed to make any response at all with the left hand. Within a month following surgery, however, Cases II and III performed the cross-localizing test for all body areas except the hands with considerable facility whereas Case I improved very little, if at all.

All patients have remained unable to perform intermanual localization tasks (Fig. 26). When the digits and palmar surface of one hand are lightly stimulated, the thumb of that hand is easily capable of pointing to the stimulated point. For example, if a series of points are stimulated on the left hand, the thumb of the left hand is able to accurately locate the point of stimulation. If the patient is required to point to the corresponding area on the opposite hand with the thumb of that hand, a dramatic inability is apparent. Thus, stimulation of the right hand, for example, finds the thumb of the left hand unable to point to the corresponding point on the left hand. This condition persists following commissurotomy.

In both early and late phases of testing, when light taps were applied doubly, i.e., at two separated points simultaneously, on opposite sides of the body, double manual responses were carried out accurately with each hand responding to the homolateral stimulus. When a subsequent verbal description of the two stimulus points was asked for, those on the left side were usually not reported. This was true even though the subject had correctly found the point of stimulation with his left hand.

TEMPERATURE DISCRIMINATION

As in early testing of cross-localization of touch, tests on thermal sensitivity showed that stimulation of the left half body below the neck, with either a warm or cool thermal probe, would not result in a correct verbal response. If a nonverbal response was requested, however, i.e., a warm or a cool stimulus was first presented and the subject was then required to match it by retrieving an object with a similar temperature from two others, he performed well. When this comparison was attempted intermanually, the response again fell to chance. Those areas on the head and face which seem to be bilaterally represented, as indicated by the tactile test, also proved to be able to relay thermal discrimination information involving either verbal or hand responses on either side.

As testing progressed, the ability of Case II and III to call out which of two stimuli presented to the left hand was hot or cold greatly improved.

PAIN SENSIBILITY

When the patients were stimulated by either a scratch or pin prick over various body regions, there appeared to be no improvement in their ability to cross-localize points of stimulation on the hands. As in the above, points stimulated over the entire right half body could be named and described, as well as points on the left half body, except for the hand.

POSITION SENSE

In tests of joint and position sense, the several joints, such as the wrist, elbow, shoulder, knee, and ankle were placed in a given position by the examiner; then the subject, wearing a blindfold, was required to state verbally the position of the relevant distal portion of the limb. This presented no problem for the right hand and foot, but the task proved difficult when the description involved the joint position of the left wrist, left fingers, and left toes (Fig. 27). Sense of position at the left shoulder, and probably also the left elbow, was preserved. Position was correctly reported without difficulty for all joints on the right arm, and also for the left knee and ankle. When the right arm was held out simultaneously with the left, however, thereby equalizing and obscuring the secondary mechanical tensions across the spinal column, ability to describe the position of the left arm dropped to chance. Also, when the end of a pencil was held in one hand and positioned by the experimenter at different angles and positions, the subject was unable to reach accurately for the other end of the pencil with the opposite hand. Taken together, this suggests that position sense is also crisply lateralized. The ability to discriminate position of the left shoulder and elbow appears due to the secondary cross-cuing effects described. When this information is intermixed and competing

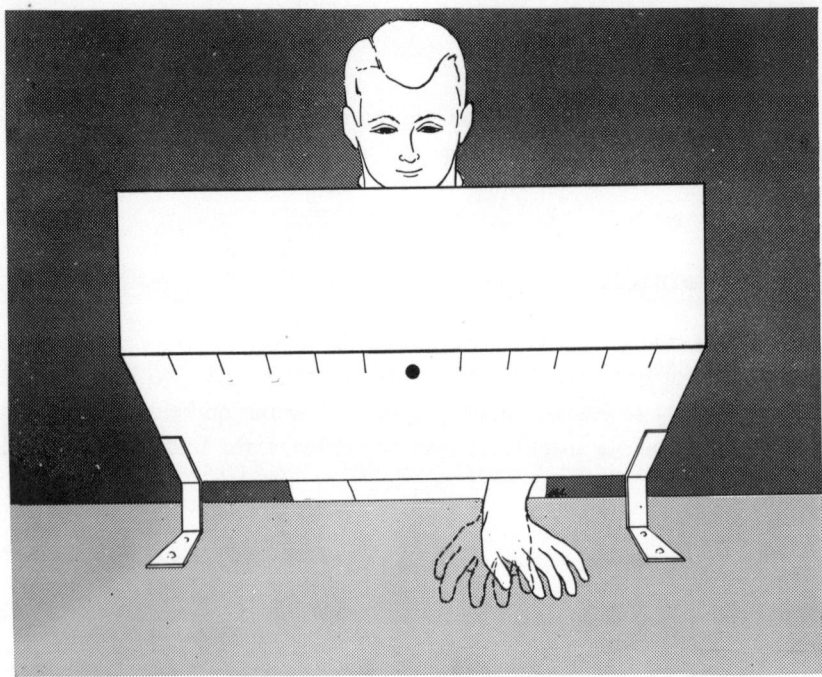

Figure 27. With left hand out of view, passive positioning of the hand by the examiner pivoted at the wrist found a split-brain patient unable to describe whether or not it was pointed to the right, to the left, or straight ahead. It is interesting to note the motor responses directed by the ipsilateral left hemisphere were accurate. This suggests position-sense information of the distal musculatures, which is projected to the right hemisphere, is not needed by the left command hemisphere in responses of this kind.

with position information concerning the right half of the body, the descriptive capacity breaks down.

PSYCHOLOGIC STUDIES

No intermanual transfer of tactile discriminations was apparent during any phase of the testing program, as long as secondary cues were limited. Tactile memory problems, where the patients on one trial learned to choose one of two stimuli, showed on the average no transfer. Test objects placed in one hand could easily be retrieved with the same hand from a grab bag containing ten objects, but not with the opposite hand. Also, simple wooden jigsaw puzzles could be put together cor-

INTERMANUAL TACTILE COMPARISON

JIGSAW PATTERN	ONE PATTERN IN EACH HAND		BOTH IN L H	BOTH IN R H
	L H	R H		
1	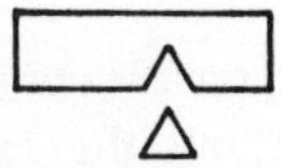 Not Completed		Correct	Correct
2 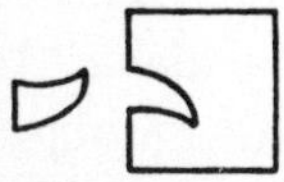	"		"	"
3 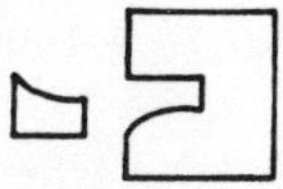	"		"	"

Figure 28. Simple jigsaw cutout puzzles could not be solved when half the information went to each hand, whereas the task was easily solved when one hand manipulated both block pairs.

rectly with either hand separately, but not when cooperation between both hands was required (Fig. 28). Contrary to the foregoing, there was complete intermanual transfer of stylus maze problems.

COMMENT

The subject's ability both to verbalize correctly the qualitative nature of somatic stimuli and to localize with accuracy, both verbally and with either hand, cutaneous stimulation on either side of the face and top and back of the head, indicates a strong ipsilateral representation of sensation for these cranial areas in both hemispheres which is equal to, or almost as efficient as, the contralateral representation.

Below the neck, the results were different. In Case I, responses to somatosensory input were made appropriately only when the main cortical motor control came from the hemisphere contralateral to stimulation. Verbal reports of stimulation confined to the left side were grossly inaccurate, and often absent, depending on the testing procedure. In Cases II and III, however, crossed responses below the neck went well for the torso and the proximal areas of the limbs. Good verbal localization was also possible for these areas. The differences between results on Cases I, II, and III may best be explained in terms of greater extracallosal brain damage apparent in Case I. Such damage might incapacitate weak secondary systems conceivably involved in ipsilateral body representation, such as, perhaps, the secondary somatosensory area.

Clearly, since the patients with more or less pure commissural lesions were able to report a considerable amount about the nature of left-sided stimulation, it seemed likely that some simple object held in the left hand might be correctly identified by the patients. In other words, the left hemisphere might be able to discriminate objects held in the left hand. This proved to be the case, as mentioned in Chapter 2. If only two objects were available for palpation, such as a round ball and a square, and the subject was informed that only these two stimuli would be used, Cases II and III performed at a high level when asked to call out which of the two had been placed in the left hand. If these same two objects were presented in series with a number of other objects and no "verbal set" was given to limit what might be presented, a poor score resulted.

Thus, it came to be seen that this kind of ipsilateral cuing mechanism allows leakage of some types of information about the nature of objects held in one hand over to the ipsilateral hemisphere. It works much more efficiently if the receiving brain is "set" and the conditions for response are limited.

The foregoing analysis has important implications for studies on cats and monkeys. Several studies have shown a certain degree of intermanual transfer of tactile discrimination in split-brain monkeys (Glickstein and Sperry, 1960; Ettlinger and Morton, 1966). Examination of the stimuli used would suggest that the same type of ipsilateral cuing mechanism might have been involved. (Indeed, in the cat and monkey, the evidence is quite clear that ipsilateral fiber systems exist.) The general importance of knowing about such strategy is, of course, that when the untrained paw of a split-brain cat or monkey can perform at a high level, one cannot conclude that interhemispheric transfer of tactile learning has occurred. Rather, it could be that either (1) both hemispheres learned the problem simultaneously even though initially the animal was trained with one hand; or, (2) that when the "untrained hand" was being tested, it queried the trained hemisphere through ipsilateral somatosensory mechanisms.

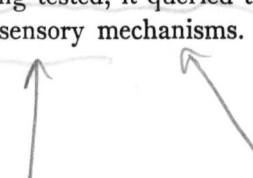

OBSERVATIONS ON AUDITORY PERCEPTIONS

In the early days of testing, only very simple tests on auditory function were carried out. In brief, in tests on auditory localization no detectable abnormalities were observed. With a patient sitting in front of a semicircle of a number of small radio speakers, brief voicing of one would result in the patient correctly localizing it with either hand or accurately describing its relative position.

In simple tests of auditory comprehension through each ear, all subjects performed with ease and accuracy. Here, stereophonic earphones were used and commands were delivered to one ear or the other with good comprehension observed under each ear condition. For example, the command to describe an auditory input presented singly to either the left or the right ear was easily done. Likewise, the command to retrieve with either the left hand (right hemisphere function) or right hand (left hemisphere function) objects named to one or the other ear presented no difficulty (Gazzaniga, 1966d, unpublished).

More recently, Milner et al. (1968), carried out tests under conditions of dichotic stimulation. Here, using Kimura's modified version of Broadbent's test, the simultaneous presentation of a series of six digits, three to each ear, found the callosum-sectioned patients unable to report with any great accuracy those presented to the left ear. These data were interpreted as being consistent with the earlier observation of Kimura (1967) that the crossed auditory pathways are more dominant than the ipsilateral projections.

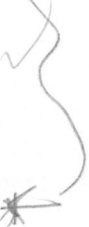

Using a similar, yet different, testing approach, Day (1969) has made a variety of fascinating findings on experienced patients LB and NG. In brief, one aspect of her test requires the subject to "fuse" the separate inputs to each ear. For example, "pahduct" is presented to one ear and "rahduct" is presented to the other. The callosum-intact normal distinctly hears the word "product" and not the nonsense antecedents. In these two split-brain patients, case LB did not hear the "fused" words. He reported only the word presented to the right ear. Case NG, however, fused rather routinely.

The finding of Milner et al. (1968) would suggest that fusion ought not to occur in commissure-sectioned patients. It clearly did in Case NG, thereby suggesting integration at some level in the auditory system. It is conceivable that the differences between Cases NG and

LB are related to a presently unknown difference in the extent of surgery.

In addition to these findings, quite striking differences were seen between the callosum-sectioned patients and normals on a temporal-order recall test. In this test, the subject is asked to write down which sound is heard first. As in the foregoing, the two different sounds are presented separately to each ear. The times range from simultaneous presentation of the two sounds to latency differences between the onset of the two of about 100 msec. Understandably, the normal person's ability to identify correctly the onset of a particular sound increases as the time between the presentation of the two increases. In the split-brain subjects, however, the ability to perform this at all is poor because of the strong right ear effect. More interesting, however, is the finding that their scores deteriorate as the lag between the onset of the two sounds increases! It is as if the memory mechanism in the commissure-sectioned patients is sorely impaired—as though under conditions of stern competition for attention, the bisected brain is not able to let secondary information "echo" or reverberate.

OBSERVATIONS ON VISUAL PERCEPTION

In tests of visual function, the aim was to determine the extent and kinds of interaction, if any, between the perceptual and mnemonic activities of the separated hemispheres, and to detect any differences in performance capacity of the right and left visual half-systems.

Exclusive projection of visual information to one or the other hemisphere was effected by presenting stimuli within either the right or left visual field while the subject fixated a central point (Fig. 29). (All stimuli presented in the left half-field thus went to the right hemisphere, and vice versa.) Inadvertent projection of test information into the wrong hemisphere, caused by eye movement away from the fixation point, was controlled by tachistoscopic presentation of the stimuli at $\frac{1}{10}$ to $\frac{1}{100}$ sec, combined with close observation of the subject's gaze.

ANALYSIS OF VISUAL FIELDS

In these tests, the subjects were seated before a table and told to fixate a central marker on a large upright screen approximately 3 feet ahead. With a fixation assured, a bright spot of light ½ inch in diame-

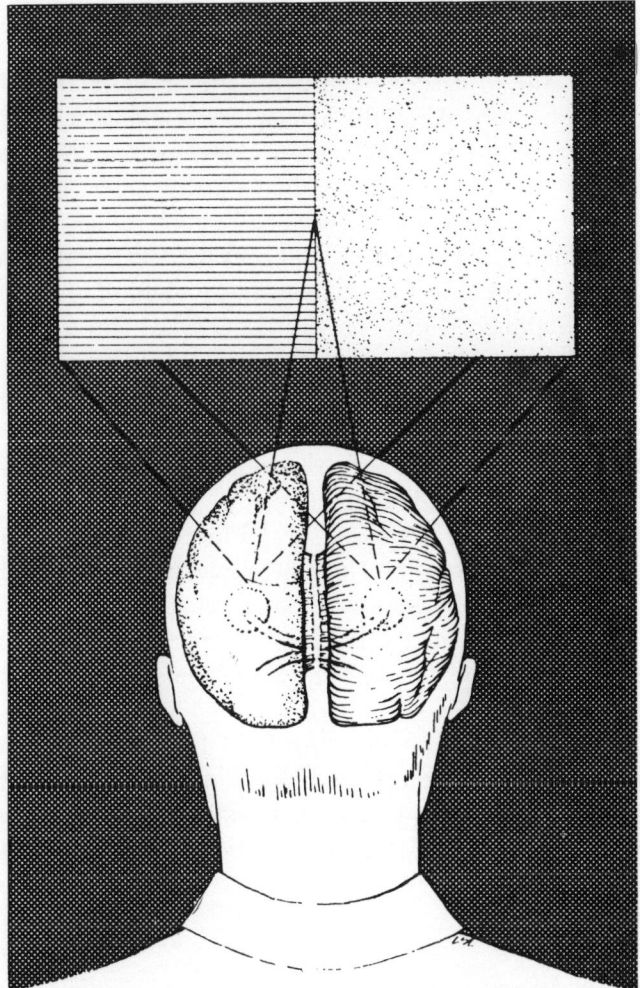

Figure 29. The left and right visual fields of man are projected to the right and left hemispheres, respectively. With the eyes held at fixation, crisp projection of information to one side of the brain or the other is easily possible.

ter was flashed in a prearranged, pseudo random schedule to different quadrants of the visual field. After each stimulus presentation, the subject was asked to describe in which quadrant the light fell. In early postoperative testing, all subjects verbally described only those lights presented in the right visual half field. Stimulation of corresponding points in the left field yielded no verbal response. When asked if they had seen anything, the subjects would claim no light had been flashed.

As both testing and recovery progressed, however, the subjects usually proved able to describe the lights presented in the left visual field. Was this because the right hemisphere could now "talk"? Was this because a subcallosal neural network became active in the interhemispheric transfer of visual information? Further analysis showed that neither of these explanations is likely to be correct; rather, it appears to be a matter of the right hemisphere cuing in the left hemisphere that a light had come on by effecting a momentary shift of gaze from the midline to the illuminated point in the visual field. Quite simply then, the left hemisphere took note that the eyes and also the head had moved and proceeded to read off where in space the eyes were oriented.

In double-field stimulation experiments, the subjects reported seeing only the light falling into the right visual field. Here, even though the lights appeared simultaneously, it seemed that the left hemisphere sets the motor system first, and its responses override those potentially emanating from the right hemisphere. Curiously, however, if each hemisphere has its own read-out mechanism, such as a push-button in the right hand for the left hemisphere, and they are therefore not competing for a common system, both hemispheres respond with equal speed.

In summary, it appears that any light falling to the left of the midline is projected to the right hemisphere, and that only light falling to the right of the midline is projected to the left hemisphere. The patients with the corpus callosum—anterior commissure sectioning seem unable to transfer visual stimuli presented to the separated hemisphere.

MACULAR SPARING

It would appear from many of the tests that the visual midline represents nothing but the abutment of the two visual fields. The visual fields were found to stop exactly in the midline, with no overlap or sparing evident. In brief, this was established by having the patients fixate a point on a rear projection screen. Small black dots ranging from two to six in number were then flashed in such a way that a certain proportion of them fell to the left of fixation, and the rest to the right of fixation. All appeared within 2° of each side of the midline. The subjects were then requested to state how many spots of light appeared on any given trial. All patients proved able to report only the dots that fell to the right of the fixation point. A dot 1 mm or more to the left of fixation went unnoticed by the left hemisphere.

STEREOPSIS

In normal man a point source of light falling in front of or behind the place of fixation can be accurately localized in depth over a range of several degrees of disparity (Westheimer and Tanzmann, 1956), and the convergent eye-movement system always knows whether to converge or diverge the eyes in order to bifixate the object. Any point in front of the plane of fixation falls on the temporal retina in both eyes and any point behind fixation falls on the nasal retina in both eyes. Therefore, in terms of the classical view of visual anatomy, the information should end up in separate hemispheres. Because of the necessity to get the disparate information together, the question becomes: Does some central strip of retina in each eye project directly to both optic tracts and therefore to both hemispheres, or does the information come together via fibers crossing in the corpus callosum, or some other brain commissure system?

This problem has been studied by Blakemore (1969); Blakemore and Mitchell (1969); and Mitchell and Westheimer (1968). Initially, they studied a young boy with a split chiasm. The subject was able to see two similar images (thin vertical slits) flashed onto the temporal retina of each eye a short distance away from the fovea, and was also able to tell that the flashed object giving rise to these two disparate images lay in front of the fixation point. In this case, the information must be arriving in the separate hemispheres; therefore, there must be some interhemispheric route for transfer of the information necessary for the brain to work out the retinal disparity.

In testing some of the split-brain patients in the present series, Blakemore and Mitchell (1969) determined that the subjects could discriminate the retinal disparities of images in the peripheral visual field (i.e., where all the information went to one hemisphere). With the fixation point off to one side, subjects were easily able to tell whether the stimulus was in front of or behind the fixation point. However, if the object was flashed directly in front of or behind the fixation point, so that images in the two eyes projected to different hemispheres, the patient could not tell whether the stimulus was nearer or farther than the plane of fixation. Therefore, it would appear that the corpus callosum serves the essential function of integration of this kind of information. Lastly, Mitchell and Westheimer looked at the question of convergent eye movements in the brain-bisected patients. Again, for disparate images flashed in the periphery, the eyes made the correct convergent or divergent response, but for images in front of or behind the fixation point the brain did not know whether to converge or diverge the eyes. Therefore, it is clear that the ocular-motor system also does not have midline disparity information in the split-brain human. All the foregoing indicates that the corpus callosum is essential for the transfer of information used in building up the input to disparity-sensitive neurons representing the region of visual space around the fixation point (Blakemore, 1969).

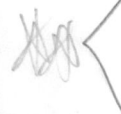

RETRIEVAL TEST FOR PATTERN DISCRIMINATION

A variety of visual-visual retrieval tests were designed in which the subject was obliged to select from a group of five figures, each on a 3 x 5-inch card placed on a table in front of him, the one that corresponded to the pattern flashed tachistoscopically on the screen. Geometric symbols, letters, numbers, pictures of objects, and single words were used. In some trials, a simultaneous verbal description was requested, while others involved only the manual response. The stimuli were flashed on the screen in either or both visual half fields on a randomized schedule, so that the subjects could not anticipate where the next stimulus would appear. The subject then tried to pick out (by pointing with the finger of one hand) from the series of five cards in front of him the pattern, picture, or word most like the projected figure.

In this situation, the right hand of all patients responded correctly with virtually 100 percent accuracy to all stimuli presented in the right field, regardless of their nature. When stimuli were presented to the left field, the left hand of Case I was able to seek out the correct card at a level 2.5 times better than chance, while Cases II and III performed almost perfectly. In cases where stimuli were presented in the left field only, the subjects when questioned would commonly deny having seen anything, and often seemed puzzled that they should be asked to pick up a card. Again, this type of puzzlement disappeared as testing progressed, and the subjects soon realized via cross-cuing mechanisms that some event had occurred (because of eye movements precipitated by the stimulus).

When stimuli were flashed simultaneously to both fields, and each hand, on request, responded to its respective stimulus, the *percentage* of correct retrieval by either the left or right hand did not drop. Nor were there other indications of perceptual distraction, conflict, or interference between the hemispheres under these conditions. Verbal recognition remained specific to right field stimuli here as before.

Intermodal transfer

As mentioned in Chapter 3, extensive testing was carried out on the extent to which patients could perform intermodal matching responses when (1) the stimulus pairs were presented to the same hemisphere, and (2) when one-half of the stimulus pair was presented to one hemisphere and one-half to the other.

In visual-tactile tests, pictures of various objects were quickly flashed to either the left or right hemisphere, and the subject was required to match them tactually by feeling a series of objects placed out of view (see Fig. 10). In tactile-visual tests, an object was first placed in one hand out of view and the subject was requested to release the object and point to the matching object presented in a visual display. To assure that no ipsilateral leakage had occurred—especially when testing the left hand (and therefore the right hemisphere)—the subjects, prior to making the visual match, were asked if they knew what was in their left hand. Since most of the objects were complex and no "set" had been established, all subjects failed to make a correct verbal identification, except in a few instances. Clearly, then, the left hemisphere had not been cued-in concerning the nature of the object, so that if the subsequent visual match was correct, one could safely conclude that the right hemisphere was responsible for the correct execution of the task.

The results were unequivocal. The dominant left hemisphere, using the right hand, performed perfectly in making intermodal visual-tactile comparisons. However, if the left hand was the responding hand to the visual stimuli presented to the left hemisphere, performance never rose above chance.

Equally good intrahemispheric intermodal comparisons were observed for the right hemisphere. Visual stimuli presented in the left visual field, such as pictures of an orange, spoon, ball, can opener, and the like, resulted in the left hand being able to easily retrieve corresponding objects through touch. If, following a correct response, the subject was asked what he had seen and retrieved, he was unable to say. "He" translates, of course, as the left hemisphere, and that *it* was unable to "say." As a result of the disconnection, it had neither seen the visual stimulus nor felt the tactile object. All of this information had been available to only the right hemisphere. It would follow, therefore, that it is incorrect to say "he" didn't know. A more correct statement is "mind-left" didn't know, but "mind-right" did. The difference is that "mind-right" can't talk about it, because it lacks a speech mechanism.

In tests such as the foregoing, truly dramatic examples of the disconnection syndrome are apparent. If, for example, a picture of an orange was flashed to the left hemisphere and a picture of an apple to the right, the left hand would retrieve an apple and the right hand an orange. Subsequently, the patient would be unable to name what had been flashed in the left field and what had been retrieved by the left hand. Or, if an apple had been flashed to the right hemisphere alone and the subject was allowed to palpate a series of items with only the right hand (with its major sensory projections going to the left hemisphere), a correct description of the flashed stimulus was never forthcoming, even if the subject happened to be holding the apple in the right hand at the time of the examiner's probe question.

On tactile-visual comparison, good performance was also observed. Of course, the dominant left speech hemisphere performed normally for the object held in the right hand. When objects were placed in the left hand, the patient was consistently unable to describe them. However, as soon as the object and the blindfold were removed, he had no trouble in pointing out the correct object seen in a chance position among six other objects of similar size.

SIMULTANEOUS DISCRIMINATORY REACTION TO DOUBLE FIELD STIMULATION

In this test, the subjects were seated in front of the apparatus pictured in Figure 30 and with both hands working together, were called upon to react to the green of a red/green stimulus presentation in the right visual field, and to make a brightness discrimination in the left field. Both before and after the subjects carried out the bimanual task, the right hand was run through a series of ten trials with single presentation of stimuli to the right field. Before each trial, the subject fixated on a center dot. The stimuli were randomly changed within each field

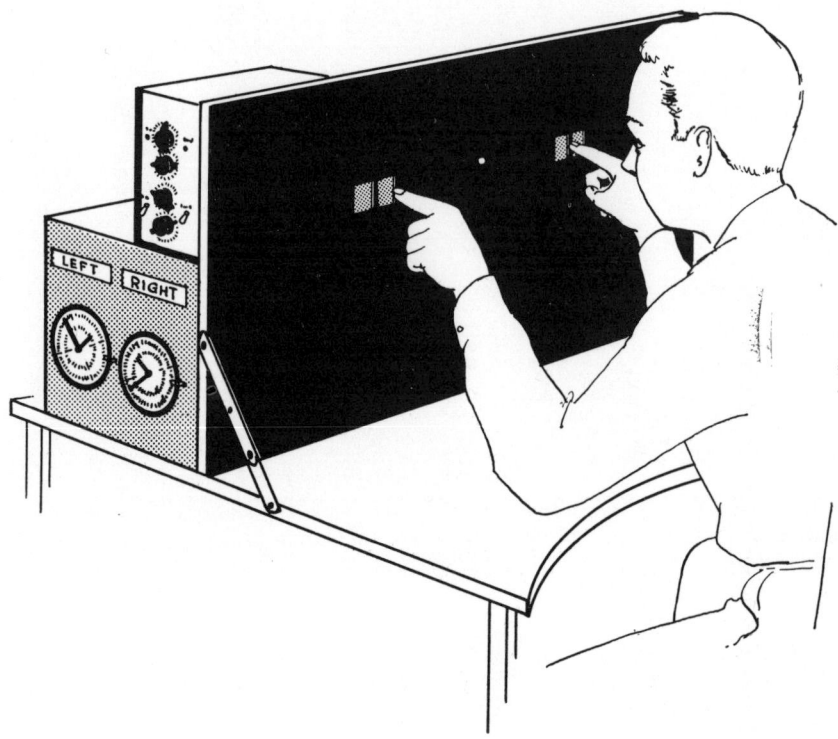

Figure 30. Apparatus to measure reaction time to visual discrimination presented either singly or simultaneously to each visual field.

from one screen to the other. The results are shown in Table 2. All cases showed consistent mean reaction times for the right hand when the second simultaneous left field discrimination was required. On the other hand, all normal controls showed significant increases in reaction time when the bimanual response was in order. However, it should be pointed out that the reaction time of both operated cases was far slower than that of the normal controls.

TESTS FOR LATERAL SPECIALIZATION OF VISUAL FUNCTION

A variety of clinical reports show that patients with right-hemisphere lesions perform worse on visual spatial tests, such as the drawing of a Necker cube, than do patients with left-hemisphere lesions

TABLE 2. Reaction Times to Visual Stimuli in Milliseconds[a].

(NORMAL AND PRE-OP.)	R. Hand (Trials 1-10)		R. Hand – L. Hand (Trials 11-20)				R. Hand (Trials 21-30)		$p(M_2-M_1)$	$p(M_2-M_4)$
	M_1	S.D.	M_2	S.D.	M_3	S.D.	M_4	S.D.		
GRN	438	57	695	97	694	96	391	56	.005	.005
TRB	465	120	770	140	800	120	496	83	.005	.005
HML	380	55	470	88	464	95	374	73	.05	.025
SRP	439	228	574	70	678	88	376	64	.005	.005
Case III	704	176	1272	213	1110	254	629	117	.005	.005
Case IV	727	158	1667	750	1227	580	682	149	.005	.005
(OPERATED)										
Case I	1150	138	869	92	798	104	848	110	N.S.	N.S.
Case II	766	156	777	153	869	224	706	280	N.S.	N.S.
Case III	705	175	724	170	741	199	582	237	N.S.	N.S.
Case IV	700	152	594	92	566	114	600	161	N.S.	N.S.

[a] R. Hand responds to red/green discrimination in right half visual field; L. Hand responds to bright/dark discrimination in left half visual field. Probability calculated from paired observations by one-tailed t-test. N.S. = 0.05

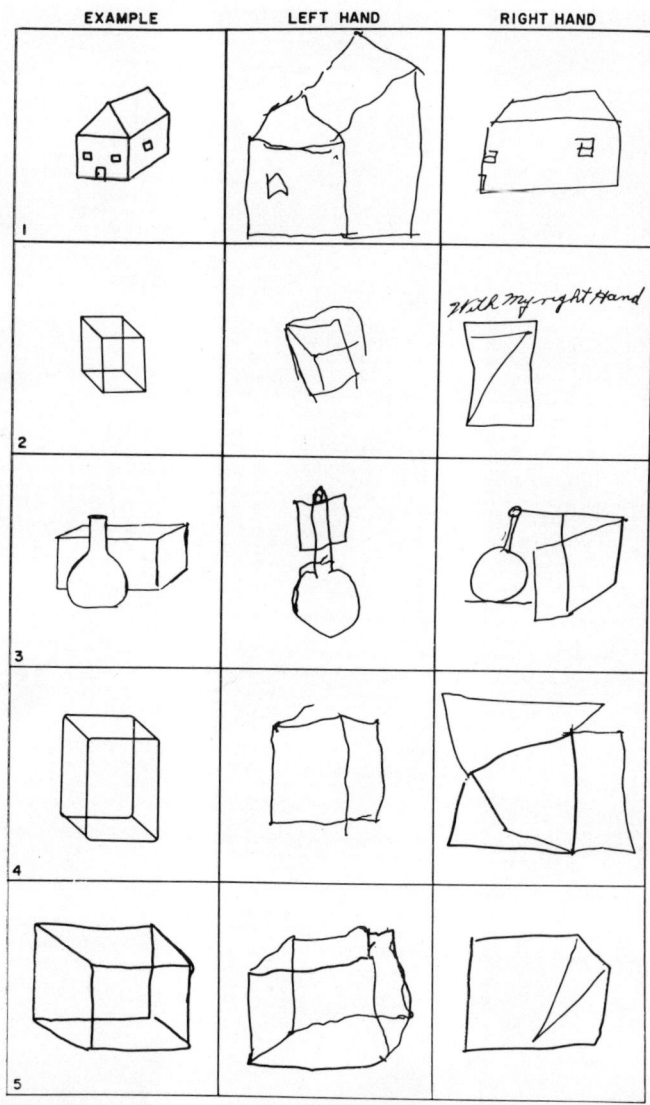

Figure 31. Representative examples of the kinds of written responses seen in Case I. These drawings were made two to three years after surgery. The left hand, which receives its major motor control from the right hemisphere, is able to draw cubes and the like, while the right hand, which is able to write, is unable to sketch these simple three dimensional designs. This phenomenon was seen in the other patients only in the first weeks or months following surgery. Because many of the other patients were essentially cases of pure commissural lesions, there was little or no problem when one hemisphere attempted to control the ipsilateral hand. The right hemisphere, which is specially built to handle this kind of task, was able to control the contralateral left arm or the ipsilateral right arm.

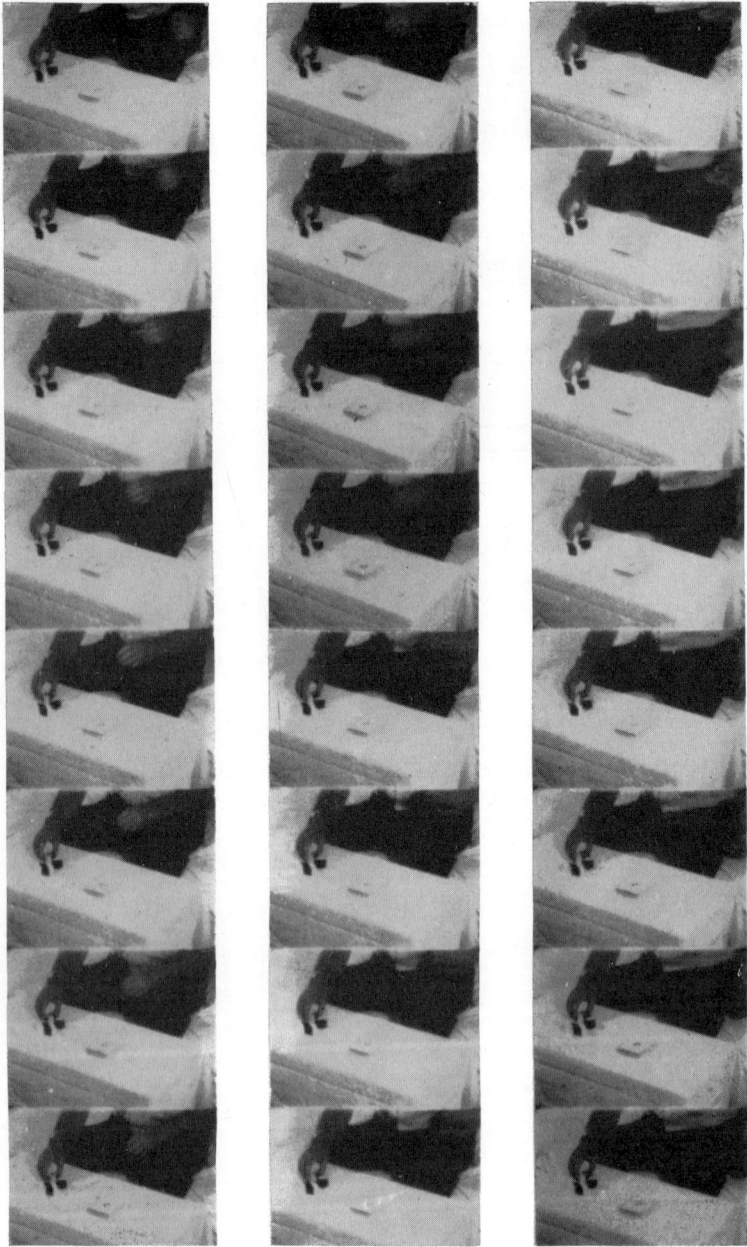

Figure 32. Case I attempts to arrange the blocks on the table to match the design on the card. The right hand was unable to carry out this task. Here, while the right hand was attempting to solve the problem, the left hand, which knows how to do the task, tries to move in and help out only to be restrained by the experimenter.

PSYCHOLOGIC AND NEUROLOGIC EFFECTS

(Bogen and Gazzaniga, 1965). In the present series of cases, we were also able to demonstrate that the right hemisphere was superior in its ability to execute this kind of test than was the left. All patients were right-handed, and they never had occasion to write or draw extensively with the left hand. Following the commissurotomy, when they copied sample figures that suggested spatial perspective like the Necker cube, their performance with the left hand was consistently better than that with the right (Fig. 31). The subjects were also able to reconstruct standard patterns in a block design test, and to assemble complex object puzzles with the left hand, but performance with the right hand was impaired (Fig. 32).

It should be noted that these observations were possible to make in only the first months following surgery in Cases II and III. In Case I, the phenomenon has persisted for eight years—it is still apparent. The reason for this is that in Cases II and III, each hemisphere quickly became equally proficient in controlling either hand. This occurred even though it was the right hemisphere which possessed the function, because of the good ipsilateral control it could effect over the right hand; hence both hands could perform at good level. In other words, the phenomenon was not observable when ipsilateral control came in. It was observable only when one hemisphere could guide and control only the contralateral hand.

INTERHEMISPHERIC MATCHING

Following callosal section, none of the patients were able to state whether two visual stimuli—one presented to the left hemisphere and one presented to the right hemisphere—were the same or different. If for example, a red spot of light was presented to the left hemisphere and a green spot to the right, no patient, by nodding his head sideways, was able to signal that the lights were different. Likewise, if both were green or both were red, no patient was able to signal that the lights were the same by nodding his head up and down. This was also true when matches were attempted on brightness problems. In other words, those remaining cerebral commissures were not able to communicate even simple visual-visual information between the two hemispheres.

No cross-integration was seen when attempts were made by the patients to tell whether or not broad lines or bars running from left to right field through the fixation point were continuous or broken at the middle. In the tests that have been done, no evidence exists that what is perceived in the right half-field has any influence on the perception or comprehension of what is seen in the left half-field.

The possibility that surgically split primates might be able to cross-compare visual information from one hemisphere to the other was first examined by Trevarthen (1963) in the monkey. In one animal, cross comparisons of circle size appeared possible. Here, a circle of a particular size was presented to one hemisphere while that of another size was presented to the opposite hemisphere. The animal was rewarded for responding to the larger of two circles. One brain-bisected animal proved able to do this. Subsequent histologic analysis confirmed the extent of surgery.

This rather remarkable finding bears close scrutiny. The question must be asked whether alternate mechanisms could possibly explain this performance rather than the subcallosal visual mechanism possibility advanced by Trevarthen (1968). In his test each hemisphere working alone could perform the problem when both stimuli were presented to it. Thus each half-brain could easily assign values to each of the five circles used. Call the largest circle Number 1, the next largest Number 2, and so on. If each hemisphere adopted the following rather simple strategy, successful performance would result. In brief, each hemisphere knows Number 1 is always correct. Whenever it appears, an immediate response is initiated by whichever hemisphere sees it and no matter what the size of the other circle. Thus, if Number 1 is projected with Number 2, the response is immediate, for each half-brain knows Number 1 is always correct, and therefore makes no attempt to compare. But what if circle Number 2 is projected with Number 3? Here, the half-brain viewing the rather large Number 2 notices its partner is not responding instantly, and therefore deduces it must not be seeing Number 1. It concludes it must be Number 3 or lower and therefore decides it is the larger and responds appropriately.

At the same time, each hemisphere knows Number 5 is always wrong. Whenever it is projected, the rule would be to immediately direct a hand to the opposite button. Thus, when Number 5 was projected with Number 4, there would be in a sense no contest for each hemisphere working alone would know to press the opposite button. When Number 4 was projected with Number 3, as in the above, each hemisphere would know to press the opposite button if it observes the opposite hemisphere didn't immediately take control and direct the hand. Any combination of circles on a five scale sequence would precipitate this state of affairs.

It is interesting to note that this notion of cooperative strategies requires two half-brains. One brain working alone could not perform at a high level. One brain seeing a Number 2 would not know if it was correct or incorrect. It only is possible for it to deduce it is correct by observing the response latency of another cooperating system.

Thus it would seem there is room for doubt that Trevarthen's animal performed the task using a subcortical visual mechanism. Recently, Hamilton et al. (1968), reported that split-brain monkeys were unable to make simple color matches when the input was divided between the two hemispheres which is consistent with an earlier finding (Hamilton & Gazzaniga 1964) that color discriminations do not transfer in the monkey. They also report one animal trained for several thousand trials was unable to do a circle size comparison task identical to the one used by Trevarthen.

In a related series of experiments Lee-Teng and Sperry (1966) reported split-brain monkeys were able to cross compare size in a tactual discrimination task so long as only five matches were used. When the tested series was extended to ten cross-comparisons, the ability completely disappeared. The data seem entirely consistent with the notion outlined above.

In man, Trevarthen (1969) reports some of the brain-bisected patients are able to match the heights of vertical bars presented separately to each half field. This kind of task could be done easily by a cooperative strategy. Slight vertical displacement of the eyes, directed by one hemisphere (a dimension not measured with the recording techniques used) would have the effect of cuing the other hemisphere as to whether the new eye position left the center of gaze at the right height. If so, the task is complete. If not, a signal for another stimulus is made by the subject and a cross match cooperative strategy recycles.

In another experiment it is claimed brain-bisected man can report through speech whether or not a stimulus falling into the left visual field is approaching or receding from the plane of fixation or moving to the right or left. Here again, using a cooperative strategy the task could easily be performed. What would seem to be a case of right hemisphere speech or of visual information cross over fades into an open question. By the simple expedient of moving the head slightly backward for an approaching stimulus (quite a normal response to a looming figure) the left speech hemisphere could deduce the direction of the stimuli's flight. Likewise a slight head deflection to the front controlled by the right hemisphere could cue the left that an object must have been receding.

Once one becomes atuned to the multiple possibilities for cross-cuing strategies, one becomes aware of the exceedingly difficult problem in designing tests to rule out these possibilities in tests of visual cross-comparisons. It is easy to think of the many ways behavioral strategies could be used by imagining being tied together with another person and imagining the number of subtle ways one could cue in the other through peripheral mechanisms as to what was going on in his own visual sphere.

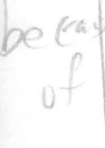

It is split-brain experiments of this kind which has led Trevarthen (1968) to argue for the existence of important mid-brain exchange mechanisms in the visual sphere. While there are undoubtedly extra-cortical mechanisms of vision (Humphrey and Weiskrantz, 1967) it would appear the split-brain studies reported to date do not as yet justify the view that mid-brain mechanisms exchange quite complex visual information.

SUMMARY

Surgical disconnection of the cerebral hemispheres produces clear-cut functional disturbances that correlate directly with the anatomic separations effected by the surgery. Activities that involve speech and writing are well preserved, insofar as they can be governed from the left hemisphere. Visual information does not transfer from one hemisphere to the other, nor is there evidence that the perceptual activities of one hemisphere influence the other, for all cases failed to achieve even the simplest sort of integration between the two visual half-fields.

One of the interesting questions regarding lateral specialization in the human cerebral cortex concerns the nature of the specialized functions allocated to the so-called minor or nondominant hemisphere. A number of studies, based mainly on patients with unilateral cortical damage, suggest that the perception of certain kinds of spatial relationships, the recognition of faces and certain nonverbal auditory functions, like timbre and tonal memory, are among those which are more highly developed in the minor hemisphere (Milner, 1962). Commissurotomy cases, in which both hemispheres remain essentially intact but separated, offer obvious advantages for the testing of such lateral specialization. To a considerable degree, the properties of each hemisphere are reflected independently in the performance of the appropriate hand, especially in the first patient and during the first months in Cases II and III. The superior performance of the left hand over the right in the block-design test, drawing, and other simple tasks that incorporate spatial relationships, observed in all patients, offers striking support that this aspect of visual activity is represented principally in the right hemisphere. Again, it would seem that the corpus callosum in the normal brain must play a critical role in serving to integrate this component of visual function with others specific to the left hemisphere.

In regard to the foregoing, it is also of interest to note that while both patients were incapable of reconstructing Necker cubes, block designs, and the like, with the right hand, they were capable of matching the test stimulus by simply pointing with this hand or indicating the correct design among a sampling of five related patterns. This shows that the primary perceptual capacity of the left, dominant, hemisphere is capable of discriminating between correct and incorrect reconstructions. Since it is also true that both patients have no motor problems with the right hand, the difficulty in reconstruction in these visual tests must lie somewhere in between these two that the lateral specialization lies more in the motor executive or expressive sphere than in the sensory-perceptual components of the performance.

Psychologic and Linguistic Characters of the Separated Hemisphere

OBSERVATIONS ON EMOTIONALITY

Of all the kinds of behavior conceivably represented in both the right and left hemispheres, one would expect to see biologically rooted emotional responses to provocative stimuli. Would the right and left hemispheres find pictures, such as pin-ups, amusing or provocative, when quickly flashed to their respective visual fields. Prior to running the experiment it was thought that some physiologic measures would be necessary, such as GSR, pupillary change, and the like. Much to our surprise, no such measures were needed. When a pin-up was flashed without warning to the right hemisphere of Case II, amongst a series of more routine stimuli, she first said, upon being asked by the examiner, that she saw nothing, but then broke into a hearty grin and chuckle (Fig. 33). When queried as to what was funny, she said

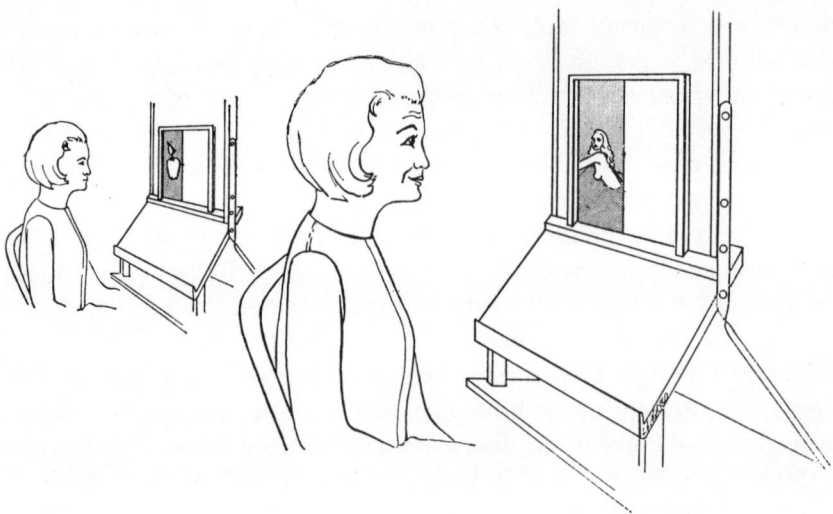

Figure 33. Nature of subject's response to both routine and provocative visual stimuli are shown. After the nude is flashed, the subject denies seeing anything and then begins to chuckle. The left speech hemisphere reads off the overall systemic changes and says something funny happened, but doesn't know what.

that she didn't know, that the "machine was funny, or something." When the picture was flashed at the left hemisphere she laughed too, and quickly reported the picture as being a nude woman. Using a different modality (olfaction), Gordon and Sperry (1968) recently confirmed this kind of result.

Neither hemisphere in Case I found the nude overtly funny (he was 51 at the time of testing), but did find other testing situations humorous. In one test of tactile learning capacity, using the left hand, Case I broke out laughing when feeling one member of a stimulus pair. The particular stimulus consisted of a tack nailed into the middle of a wooden square block. Every time he felt it, he would pick it up and twirl the block about the axis and would chuckle heartily when doing so. When asked what was funny he would say, "I don't know, something in my left hand I guess."

Because of the aforementioned apraxia of Case I, whereby good control for a particular hand was forthcoming only when commands were coming from the contralateral hemisphere, severe problems in unitary action sometimes occurred. In the other cases, where the will and intent of one hemisphere (and usually the left) could prevail over the entire motor system, antagonistic behavior between the two halves of the body was kept at a minimum. Case I, however, would sometimes find himself pulling his pants down with one hand and pulling them up with the other. Once, he grabbed his wife with his left hand and shook her violently, while with the right trying to come to his wife's aid in bringing the left belligerent hand under control. Once, while I was playing horseshoes with the patient in his backyard, he happened to pick up an axe leaning against the house with his left hand. Because it was entirely likely that the more aggressive right hemisphere might be in control, I discretely left the scene—not wanting to be the victim for the test case of which half-brain does society punish or execute.

Case III was judged to be too young to be exposed to the livelier aspects of our slide collection. He, nevertheless, clearly showed these same kinds of phenomena. Because of his good ability to understand spoken words in the right hemisphere (see below) he would consistently show the following kinds of reactions. After either a red or a green light was flashed to the right hemisphere, the patient was asked to guess the color; performance was at a chance level, as might be expected if the speech mechanism is solely represented in the left hemisphere. After a few trials, however, the score improved whenever the examiner allowed a second guess. We discovered that what was occurring was that if a red light was flashed, and the patient, by chance, guessed red, he would stick with that answer. If the flashed light was red and the patient, by chance, guessed green, he would frown, shake his head and say, "Oh no, I meant red." Our interpretation is that the right hemisphere saw the light, heard the left hemisphere make the guess green, and knowing the answer was wrong, the right hemisphere precipitated the frown and a shake of the head, which in turn cued-in the left hemisphere to the fact that the answer was wrong and that it had better correct itself. In addition to the foregoing, there is strong evidence that not only humorous responses can be precipitated, but also emotional responses resembling displeasure with stimuli or more directly displeasure with one's own behavior. Similar observations have been made in the monkey (Fig. 34).

It would appear, then, that the right hemisphere as well as the left hemisphere can emote, and while the left can tell you why, the right cannot. Because the right hemisphere precipitated a gross response most likely involving neural, humoral, and autonomic changes as well as muscular changes, and so forth, the left hemisphere is cued-in to the fact that something has happened. It is, however, unable to get at the cognitive aspects of whatever produced the emotional change. This

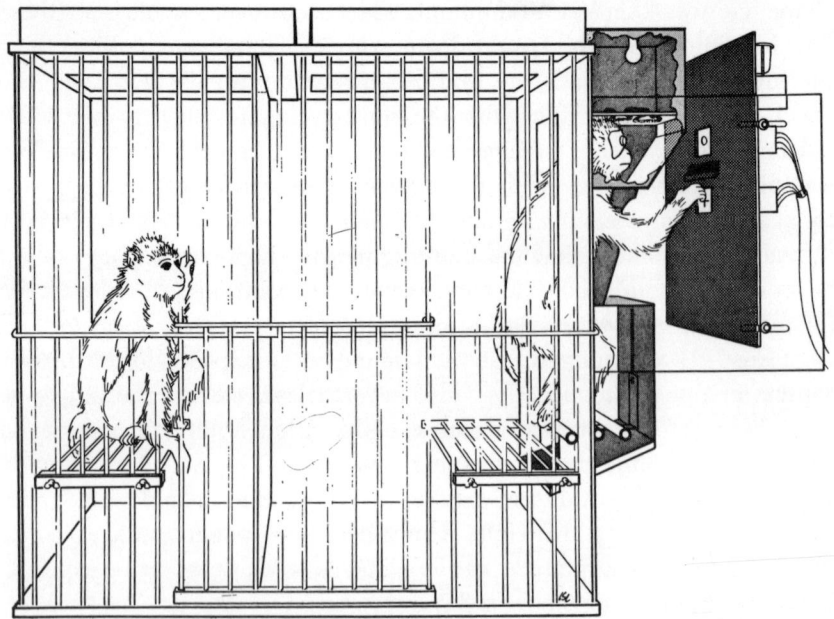

Figure 34. Split-brain monkeys permanently fitted with goggles equipped with a red filter over one eye and a blue filter over the other were placed in a specially designed testing apparatus, which could be illuminated by either a red or blue light. They were trained and maintained in blue light, thereby allowing vision through only the eye covered with the blue filter. Under these conditions other visual stimuli were briefly presented to the opposite hemisphere in red light. Stimuli with emotional quality presented in this manner were distractive and could affect the normal performance of the ongoing activity of the opposite working hemisphere. Additionally, if a fear-producing stimulus was directly presented to a hemisphere while it was engaged in some visuomotor task, immediate testing of the opposite hemisphere showed it to be relatively undisturbed provided the exposure was brief. With protracted exposure, the animal's behavior was found to be equally disturbed in each hemisphere. Testing and training apparatus used throughout all experimentation is shown above. Color of room environment as well as stimulus patterns on response panel could be changed from red to blue by remote control.

observation is in basic agreement with the fascinating experiment of Schachter (1967). He administered epinephrine to normal subjects in order to increase their state of arousal. The test situation was such that the subjects did not know why they felt different and as a consequence eagerly searched for cues from the environment to explain their state. Subjects exposed to positive, cheerful cues explained how happy they felt, while subjects exposed to negative adversive cues claimed they felt depressed. This neo-James-Lange finding is in accord with

OBSERVATIONS ON INTELLECTUAL FUNCTIONS

To date, the experimental procedures used in testing the split-brain patients has precluded an extensive evaluation of the intellectual functions of the separated hemispheres. While nonverbal I.Q. tests exist (e.g., Raven's Progressive Matrices), proper administration is extremely difficult because of the need for prolonged exposure of test stimuli. This, as mentioned earlier, cannot easily be done because of the need of a tachistoscopic method of presentation of stimuli in order to avoid eye movements. Nonetheless, the problem is of considerable interest, and the sparse data that do exist should be examined.

In fairness to the right hemisphere, all tests require nonverbal responses. Using the simplest test imaginable, patients were required to respond by pushing the appropriate button of a discriminandum to the red of a red-green stimulus pair, or the "plus" of a "plus-zero" pattern discrimination when presented to either the left or right hemisphere. The reinforcement was a click, information that both hemispheres had received. In order to rule out the possibility of stimulus preference, the first response on the initial trial was usually not rewarded. In all patients tested, this task was quickly learned by either hemisphere. In transfer tests, each half-brain worked independently and separately, since no interaction or carryover was observed. When the right hemisphere was responding perfectly, for example, the left was completely unable to describe the two stimuli being discriminated.

More recently, J. D. Johnson and I (1969) looked at the question of whether a lateralized reinforcement cue to the hemisphere not receiving the stimulus would hinder learning. In this test, the patient had to respond to the "one" of a "one-zero" discrimination presented solely to the right hemisphere. As soon as the response was made, either the word "right" or "wrong" would appear in the opposite visual field, thereby being exclusively projected to the left hemisphere. When the situation remained rather academic, the patient, after 30 trials, had failed to learn the problem! But, if both the stimulus and the reply were projected to either side alone, the discrimination was learned in one or two trials.

In contrast to the above, if an incorrect response in the split field condition is accompanied by secondary cues, learning is evident. In this case, prior to the test, the patient was admonished for performing so poorly on the previous 30 trials. Case II was told in aggressive terms that the test was extremely easy and that anyone should be able to perform the task. She said she would try especially hard on the next test. Subsequently, on the first trial she responded in error, which resulted in the "wrong" sign appearing. She frowned, shook her head in disgust, and sighed. On the next trial the same thing occurred. On the third trial she was correct, and from then on never made an error.

In the parlance of brain circuitry, it would appear that as long as the reward signal remained "cool" or cortical, the split brain was unable to put the information together with the appropriate stimulus. It is the cortical-cortical connections which are severed in cerebral commissurotomy. If, on the other hand, the "cool" stimulus precipitates a more general systemic response, the effects of which can be monitored by the opposite hemisphere, learning results. It is as if a variety of reinforcement mechanisms exist with respect to brain circuitry, each signaling the system about the environment, but that information with greater arousal value produces a more general and diffuse response.

Reversal learning on simple tasks appears possible in each separate hemisphere. Both tactual and visual stimuli, once learned, can easily be reversed, with equivalent scores seen for each hemisphere. Some question remains, however, whether the right hemisphere is capable of carrying out extradimensional shifts.

In an attempt to ascertain whether the same kinds of mental processes were active in the solution of simple problems in each hemisphere, pupillary responses during a match to sample tactile discrimination were monitored (Fig. 35). The patients were seated in front of a closed-circuit video tape camera equipped with a magnifying lens which allowed for a sharp, crisp, large image of the pupil. Tactile objects varying along one dimension, namely shape, were presented to either the left or the right hand, which means (because of the care used in choosing the stimuli) that the right or left hemisphere perceive, exclusively, the stereognostic components. Specifically, when the pupil appeared stable, an object was placed in one hand and the subject palpated it for a few seconds. The object was then withdrawn, followed by an inactive period, and then another object was presented. The patient was then required to make a match. As can be seen in Figure 35, the pupil dilated at the "storing" stage, and also dilated at the "retrieval" stage of the task, with no apparent differences evident for

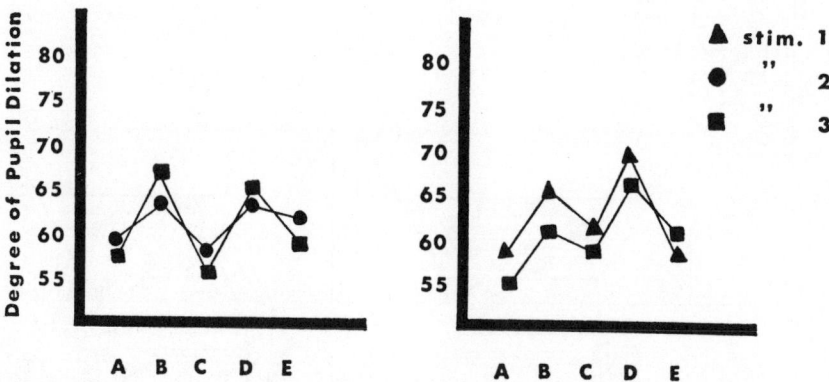

Figure 35. Course of pupil dilation in case L.B. (Case III) when: A, resting; B, sampling tactile stimulus; C, waiting (30 seconds); D, searching for match; E, resting. Case N.G. (Case II) showed similar responses, and neither patient showed a difference for left or right hands.

either hand. This would suggest that in problems of this order, similar or identical processes were active in both the left and right hemispheres.

The foregoing studies raise new questions regarding the nature, overall capacity, and distribution of information processing systems in the primate brain. In brief, from an information processing point of view, the question becomes: Can the two hemispheres, working separately but simultaneously, perform at a higher level than the joined hemispheres of commissure-intact controls?

Experiments on this question to date have been carried out in the monkey (Gazzaniga and Young, 1967). Normal monkeys, when required to push the lit button of a pair, can handle up to six pairs—three in each visual field, after the cue lights have been left on for 600 msec. If the stimuli are presented for less time, however, their performance deteriorates. Split-brain monkeys quickly exceed this limit, and are able to respond correctly to eight pairs of lights left on for only 200 msec. (Fig. 36). Thus, the upper limit of a normal animal was surpassed following brain bisection. Similar effects have been recently observed in a related test carried out in commissure-sectioned man.

Both the patients and the controls were seated in front of a Dodge tachistoscope, and were asked to fixate a point in the center of the visual field (Fig. 37). An array of alphabetic letters were flashed

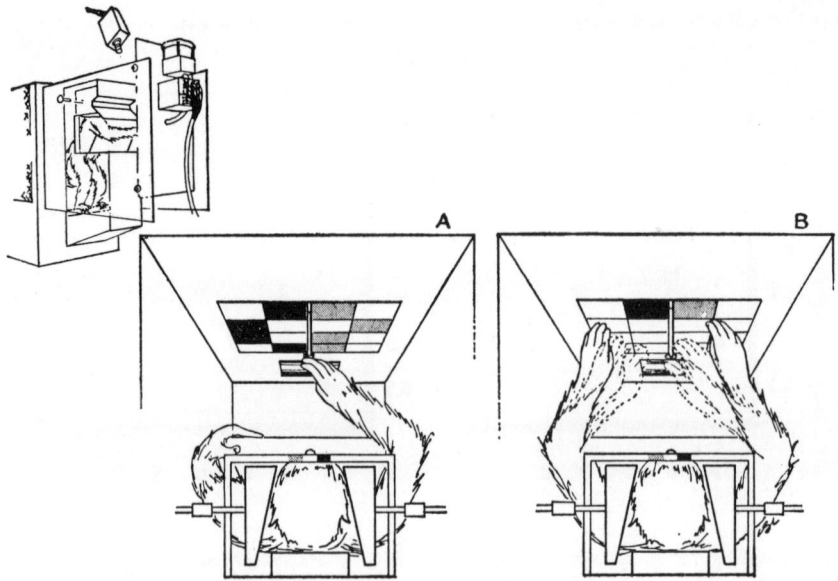

Figure 36. Split-brain monkeys can handle more visual information than normal animals. A. When the monkey pulls a knob, 8 of the 16 panels light momentarily. B. The monkey must then start at the bottom and punch the lights that were lit and no others. With the panels lit for 600 milliseconds, normal monkeys get up to the third row from the bottom before forgetting which panels were lit. Split-brain monkeys complete the entire task with the panels lit only 200 miliseconds. The monkeys look at the panels through filters; since the optic chiasm is cut in these animals, the filters allow each hemisphere to see the colored panels on one side only.

either to the left or right of fixation, or both, depending on the test condition. After presentation of the stimulus, the subject was shown a list of 20 consonants and was required to point with his left hand to as many of the test letters as could be remembered.

Prior to the test, two practice trials were run; one trial presented four vowels to the left field and one presented four vowels to the right field. On the following ten trials, the test stimuli were four black letters printed on a white background and were presented tachistoscopically for 100 msec. On half of the trials the four letters fell to the left of fixation and were therefore projected to the right hemisphere. On the other trials, the four letters fell to the right of fixation and were therefore projected to the left hemisphere. The letters were selected from 20 consonants, and each consonant appeared twice, once in the left visual field and once in the right. On each of the next ten trials,

PSYCHOLOGIC AND NEUROLOGIC EFFECTS

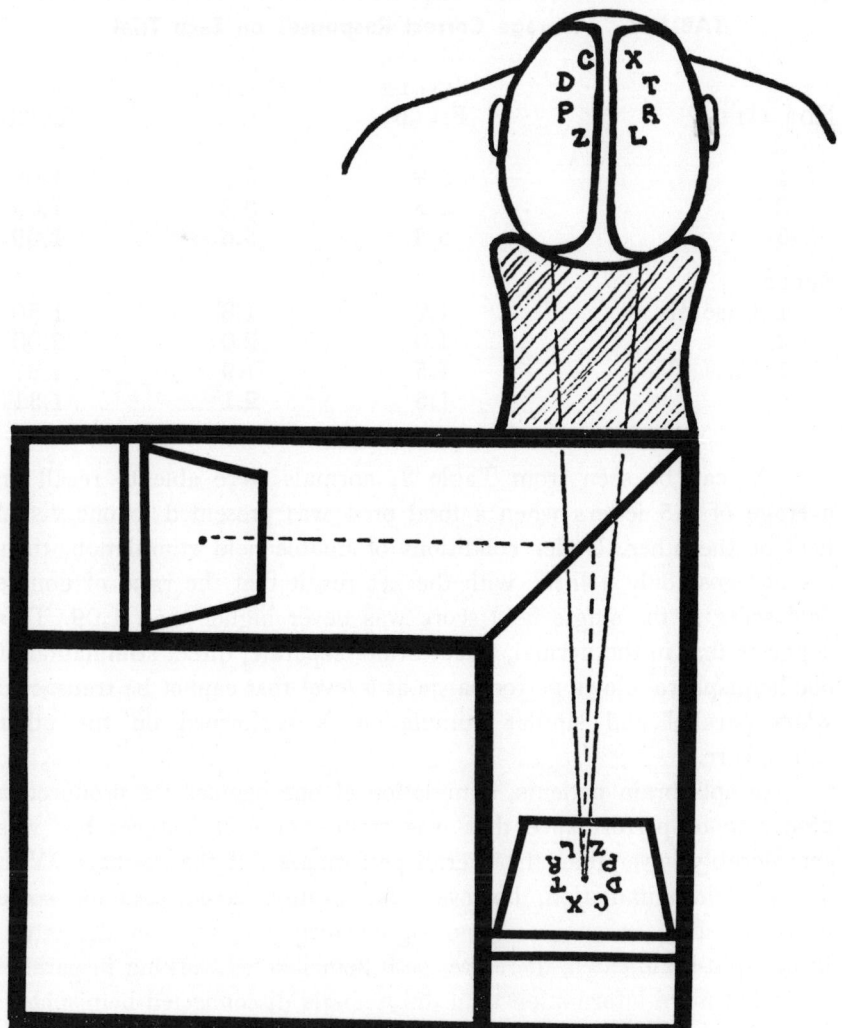

Figure 37. Schematic view of Dodge Tachistoscope, which allows constant field illumination and quick flash presentation of letters to one or both visual fields. Letters falling to the left of fixation are projected to the right hemisphere and those to the right project to the left hemisphere.

eight consonants were flashed, four in each half field. In this series, each consonant was used four times, twice on the left and twice on the right. Since the total number of responses was not limited, the error rate and rational guessing probabilities were used to correct the scores for guessing. The two patients went through the task twice, once in the sequence described above and once in reverse order.

TABLE 3. Average Correct Responses on Each Trial.

NORMALS	SINGLE FIELD	DOUBLE FIELD	RATIO
1	3.8	3.9	1.03
2	3.5	3.8	1.09
3	3.3	3.6	1.09
SPLITS			
1 Case II	1.2	1.8	1.50
2	1.0	2.0	2.00
1 Case IV	1.5	1.9	1.27
2	1.6	2.1	1.31

As can be seen from Table 3, normals were able to recall an average of 3.5 letters when a total of 4 was presented to one visual field or the other. Under conditions of double field stimulation, their average rose only a little, with the net result that the ratio of double field score to the single field score was never higher than 1.09. This suggests that in the normal, intact brain, separate, direct stimulation of one hemisphere allows performance at a level that cannot be transacted when parallel and similar stimulation is performed on the other hemisphere.

In split-brain patients, stimulation of one hemisphere produced a base rate of performance that was stable for each subject but was considerably lower than the overall performance of the normals. With double field stimulation, however, the brain-bisected patients' score nearly doubled in one case and significantly increased in the other. In the split-brain cases, therefore, both hemispheres working in parallel processed more information than did a single disconnected hemisphere. Why the split-brain subjects performed at an overall lower level than the practiced normals is not clear. A likely explanation would be that each patient had been for a number of years on anticonvulsant medication. Additionally, they were epileptic and had suffered from a certain degree of brain damage.

Inspection of the individual responses made relative to the separate hemispheres revealed that Case III reported twice as many letters projected to the left hemisphere as to the right, whereas Case II reported equally well from each hemisphere. Also, during double field stimulation, Case III always produced the left hemisphere information before the right, as well as reporting more from the left. Case II, however, using the left hand in response, always reported the right hemisphere information first, although each hemisphere performed equally well. These data on Case II are consistent with experimental studies on the monkey, which show that discrimination learning is better in the hemisphere contralateral to the responding arm (Trevarthen, 1962). This type of explanation may also hold for Case III. For weeks prior to this test, his school teacher had required him to write with his right hand hundreds of short sentences. In effect, this may have created a strong left hemisphere set, which would explain his superior scores on the left side at the expense of those on the right.

The foregoing suggests that the corpus callosum inhibits the short-term memory mechanism of each hemisphere. One possible explanation for this would be the following: In the normal, intact brain, the left speech hemisphere is aware of and can describe all aspects of the left visual field, in addition to the right field. This may not be because a duplicate pattern of the visual world is sent across via the callosum, as recent electrophysiological work described in Chapter 4 would suggest, but rather because the callosum relayed abstracted and descriptive information about that part of the visual world. It is the right hemisphere which is conscious of the left visual field, the left hemisphere being aware of the left field only as a result of the running description given to it by the right hemisphere. It is as if two people were looking at two different aspects of a similar visual scene. One could be aware of the other only indirectly by listening to a description of it, not by actually seeing it.

If this kind of informational exchange is incessantly taking place in the callosal-intact brain, the informational load placed on one hemisphere would instantly be communicated and processed in the other, leaving little channel space for more incoming information. If the hemispheres were disconnected, however, each system would be free of the job of keeping the other up-to-date, as well as listening to the other, and thereby be free to work to full capacity and in parallel with the opposite half-brain.

At the same time, caution must be exercised in the interpretation that two half-brains are better than one. Milner (1968) claims hemispherectomy in early life results in overall intellectual impairments. The impairment, however, is one of degree—such patients are not half as intelligent or the like. Recently, Sechzer (1968) claimed that split-brain cats show impairments in learning that are not seen in the normal, intact animal.

OBSERVATIONS ON SPEECH AND LANGUAGE FUNCTION

As evident from the foregoing, each hemisphere in man has visual and tactile perceptual capacities, as well as learning capabilities. Functions such as primary motor control of the speech musculature are also present in each half-brain, but the neural organization required for spoken language is usually lateralized to one cerebral hemisphere. At the same time, however, the degree of lateralization of the basic symbolic processes and engrams involved in language has been the subject of much disagreement and speculation. The question becomes: Is language present in both hemispheres, while the capacity to speak is present in one, or is language lateralized to the same degree as the speech mechanism subserving it? Some authors maintain that the engrams involved in language are laid down bilaterally (Zangwill, 1964), whereas other restrict them to areas in the left hemisphere (Penfield and Roberts, 1959).

Separation of the hemispheres offers a unique means of investigating such questions, and the results of a series of appropriate psychologic tests, in general, indicate that language function and comprehension can exist in both hemispheres, but that the ability to communicate by either written or verbal reports appears limited to the left hemisphere.

LANGUAGE EXPRESSION

Left Hemisphere

In tests aimed to determine the capacity to speak with reference to information specifically lateralized to one or the other hemisphere, very different results were obtained for the right and left sides. Spoken descriptions of stimulus material and other verbal responses, obtained from the left hemisphere, showed from the beginning little or no impairment. For example, visual stimuli such as numbers, letters, words, and pictorial material presented tachistoscopically in the right visual half field at 0.1 second were reported correctly and described normally. The same was true for stimuli presented to the right hand with vision excluded. In short, any sensory information entering the left hemisphere, or the results of the central processing of that information, could be reported through speech in much the usual manner.

Right Hemisphere

No subjects were able to give accurate spoken reports for even the simplest kind of sensory information projected to the right hemisphere. In contrast to their preoperative responses, tactual stimuli presented to the left hand or visual stimuli to the left half of the visual field evoked in each case only irrelevant confabulatory spoken responses or none at all. For example, a pencil placed in the left hand might go unnoticed and elicit no verbal comment whatever; or, more typically, its presence would be recognized, but it would be called a "can opener" or a "cigarette lighter," or whatever. Such guesses came presumably from the left dominant hemisphere, and were based on whatever indirect cues happened to be available to that hemisphere. All visual stimuli flashed to the left half field similarly went undescribed or were reported vocally as just a "flash" or a "white flash."

Month after month of testing the right hemisphere alone revealed it to be mute. Except for isolated cases reported in the literature this appeared consistent with other clinical findings. Occasionally left-hemisphere-damaged patients are reported to get off short profane bursts when highly aroused (Falconer, 1967). Smith (1966) also reports a case where left hemispherectomy did not permanently impair speech and language function.

Recently Butler and Norrsell (1968) reported that in Case III of the present series the possibility existed that speech was elicited from the right hemisphere. According to their report such words as "cup," "clap," "six," and so on, were spoken if the subject was allowed a greater viewing time of the stimulus. Using an ocular recording technique which signaled an electronic shutter to shut off a projector when saccadic eye movement occurred, they felt confident that vision had been limited to one hemisphere for a prolonged period of time. While the actual scores were not reported, the authors stated that the subject fairly reliably described a number of the stimuli. They offer a word of caution because it was not shown prior to the response, which they assumed to come from the right hemisphere, that the left was ignorant of the nature of the stimulus.

There are a number of possible explanations for the data. If the patients instead of fixating at the plane of the projection screen imagined a point a few feet or so beyond, the net effect would be to bring into the right good field of vision information that, if the subject had fixated at the plane of the screen, would have been projected exclusively to the right hemisphere. Looking "wall-eyed" in this fashion would not be picked up by the recording technique used. And, of course, there is a high payoff for the subject to develop such a strategy of diverging the eyes.

In some recent tests with the same case, S. A. Hillyard and I noticed during the course of an examination that the subject seemed able to verbally respond correctly to whether a "1" or a "0" had been flashed to the right hemisphere. When asked how he knew, the subject said, "The '0' doesn't look like an '0'; it looks like two bars of light whereas the '1' has of course but one." Here again it was not possible to rule out possible wall-eyed effects but they seemed unlikely because the stimulus light was placed far out into the periphery.

A more likely explanation for this latter observation is that simple aspects of the visual display can transfer over to the left speech hemisphere through the midbrain. Indeed, if it were the right hemisphere talking, it is most unlikely that it could carry out the detailed analysis given on why it knew it was an "0." Could it be that the midbrain leaks across stimulus primitives after a certain period of time from surgery? It is a most interesting possibility and one that merits further investigation.

Writing

The right hand, with its main motor control centered in the left hemisphere, was always capable of writing correctly the names and descriptions of visual or tactile stimuli presented to the left hemisphere, with no special difficulty evident. When the same stimulus material was presented to the right hemisphere, however, none of the stimuli could be described or named in writing by any of the patients using either hand. For example, when a spoon or a knife was placed in the left hand, or a picture flashed to the left visual field, any written responses seemed to represent mere guesswork by the major hemisphere. Writing to dictation posed no problem for these persons when they were using the right hand.

Some simple writing to dictation was possible with the left hand also after the seventh month in Case II, and after the first month in Case III, but not at all in Case I. This performance with the left hand seems best ascribed to bilaterality in motor control.

LANGUAGE COMPREHENSION

The question of the extent to which language is represented in the subordinate hemisphere has long been a matter of controversy, with authoritative proponents supporting both sides of this issue. Since no deficits are observable in the left hemisphere when tested separately, the question remained whether the minor right hemisphere is capable of some recognition and comprehension of language and other symbolic information. To investigate this possibility, we applied tests that were designed to separate the comprehension of language from its expression. The motor activity in this case was nonverbal, and depended in most instances upon pointing with the left hand to a correct answer presented as one item among an array of incorrect items. These tests failed to reveal any significant language comprehension in the damaged right hemisphere of Case I. In at least three other cases in which prior brain damage had been minimal, however, it was possible to demonstrate comprehension of verbal and other symbolic material. In general, tests utilizing visual presentations will be emphasized, since this is the only input system that allows no leakage of information to one hemisphere when visual presentation has been made to the other.

Visual Comprehension

In all tests, the subject was usually allowed to view the words and pictures to be flashed under prolonged exposure, and was asked to identify each. Subsequently, the test stimuli were quickly flashed to the separated hemispheres on a random basis, and the subjects were required to point to a word or picture that best matched the flashed stimulus. Using this test procedure, both Cases II and III proved to be capable of reading letters, numbers, and short words in the left visual field. In general, best performance was seen when the subjects were processing nominal material, and more specifically noun-object words. Adjectives were second best comprehended, and there was no evidence that verbs were understood or comprehended at all. The evidence then is as follows.

Noun Structure

In early testing, when the names of familiar objects were flashed at 0.1 second to the left field, the subject, while unable to give a correct verbal response, was nevertheless able to retrieve the matching item from among a series of ten stimuli laid in open view in front of him. If words such as knife, pen, orange, or the like, were tachistoscopically presented in the left visual field, the patients could also readily point out the correct one from among ten items arranged in free view before him. Similarly, if a picture, for example, of a "house," was flashed into the left visual field, the subjects would verbally deny having seen anything when asked. Upon being urged to let the left hand try, however, they would then proceed to pick up the card with "house" printed on it from a series laid out in open view in front of them.

The question immediately arises whether all classes of nouns are present in the right hemisphere. From unpublished studies carried out by Arthur Schwartz and myself, there is now clear evidence that nouns derived from verbs are not represented in the right hemisphere. In the extreme case when "fall," or "hit," or "jump" are used as nouns, all patients were unable to process the words meaningfully. More interestingly, "-er' nouns such as "locker," "teller," and "tropper" were not present in the right hemisphere's lexicon, whereas "-er' nouns such as "butter," "letter," "water," and "flower" were easily recognized. These data allow at least two hypotheses. First, it cannot be concluded that only noun-object type nouns are present in the right hemisphere, whereas nouns probably derived from verbs are not represented. On the other hand, good or bad performance with nouns may be solely related to the morphemic content of the word. Clearly, words like "butter" and "letter" have but one morpheme whereas agent words like "locker" and "trooper" have two.

Adjectives

Using the testing procedure described above it was also determined that the right hemisphere handles adjectives of a certain kind. When pictures of various objects were flashed to the right hemisphere, the subjects proved able to correctly identify a dominant characteristic of the stimulus. For example, when a picture of a steaming cup of coffee was flashed to the right half-brain, the subject would point to the card with "hot' printed on it from a series of other cards placed in full view. When tested in this fashion, pictures depicting a feature such as "hot," "cold," "round," and so forth, were easily identified by the right hemisphere. On the other hand, adjectives such as "shiny," "leaky," "dried,' and the like, were not handled correctly by the right hemisphere in early testing sessions. With several corrective trials, however, Cases II and III turned in a better performance.

Verbs—Printed Commands

In tests specifically aimed at the question of whether volitional actions can be triggered by verbal commands presented exclusively to the right hemisphere, simple verbs were tachistoscopically presented in the left visual field. One series required the patients to make appropriate facial responses to words like "smile," "laugh," "nod," "frown," "chew," and so on, which involved the motor system that has bilateral representation in each hemisphere. In another series, the patient was required to move the left or right hand appropriately to commands like "tap," "squeeze," "point," "knock," and so on. In all such tests, the patients displayed almost complete inability to make appropriate responses to these simple commands. Further tests indicated that the difficulty was not in making the required movement but rather in comprehension of the words. If, instead of presenting the word "knock," a picture of the same gesture was flashed to the right hemisphere, there was no problem in using the left hand to make the given movement. Further, when the test required that the left hand be used merely to point to a picture from among a series portraying the flashed word such as "knock," the performance level was poor. Inability to perform this type of task, which was readily carried out when object nouns were used, suggests that this category of language is represented poorly if at all in the right hemisphere.

Comprehension of Spoken Words

Because of the bilaterality of the auditory afferent projection, tests with the comprehension of words presented audibly to the right hemisphere were run, not by trying to lateralize the original input, but rather by limiting the available answers exclusively to the right hemisphere. In one test, the patients were required to push a response button held in the left hand when they saw one of a series of five nouns projected in serial succession to the left visual field that matched the test word spoken previously. They were able to do this, and also to pick out the correct word from a series presented to the left half field that fitted a descriptive phrase read aloud by the examiner. For example, the examiner would read "used to tell time" and would then flash five choice words in succession to the left visual field. In this instance, the patient made a correct manual sign to the word "clock." When one of them was asked in passing what word he had seen, the reply from the major hemisphere was "watch." Here, again, was another demonstration of what was constantly encountered in testing these patients; namely, complete agnosia in one hemisphere for ongoing cognitive experiences in the other hemisphere. In the foregoing, exclusive visual projection of the test material to the right hemisphere ruled out any possibility that the left dominant hemisphere played a role in determining the answer. In our original test, we also thought that presentation of stimuli to the left hand would clearly limit the input to only the right hemisphere. While this is largely true, certain "primitives" of the stimulus described in Chapter 2 do leak over to the left hemisphere, and if the left hemisphere is searching for an answer too, as is always the case with auditory input, the ipsilateral information may be sufficient for correct identification. As a result, inferences about the ability of the right hemisphere to comprehend speech as indicated by tactual retrieval tests must be looked upon with caution.

Comprehension Through Stereognosis

Because of the problem uncovered in using touch as an input channel, the results on stereognostic recognition and language are somewhat equivocal. Additionally, in all patients, as testing progressed, their sophistication and expertise in handling the examinations increased, and strategies that were sometimes seen in the early months of testing, whereby one hemisphere would cue-in the other to an answer, became practiced and routine, and were efficiently used in later months. These cross-cuing tricks are now a real problem, and at present the most stringent controls must be run before one can say that a particular hemisphere working alone does or does not possess a particular ability.

It is in tests where the left as well as the right hemisphere are exposed to the question, or where both have free access to the answer, that problems arise. For example, when an object was placed in the left hand and the subject was asked to name it, all patients consistently failed. When, however, the subject was told that the object was one of five things, or that there were five printed cards in free view in front of the subject, one of which correctly described the object, then their ability to name the object was good. Is this because the right hemisphere comprehends, or because the left hemisphere receives enough of the "primitives" of the stimulus through the ipsilateral leakage to come up with the answer? Since the latter possibility is real, this particular kind of test must be viewed with caution as an examination that demonstrates linguistic competence in the right hemisphere.

When touch is used, the only completely safe experimental situation occurs when the stimuli to be matched are presented exclusively to one hemisphere; that is, when the linguistic cues for comprehension and retrieval by stereognosis are flashed tachistoscopically to the left visual half field. Only simple, short, usually single words can be used for this form of presentation. The words are printed vertically in some cases and horizontally in others and are presented near the vertical midline of the left side in order to utilize central vision as much as possible. After correctly retrieving the objects described in the flash, the patients were asked what the item was, while the item was still in the left hand, but out of sight behind the screen. If the items were named correctly, which happened rarely, the trial was thrown out on the supposition that the eyes had probably moved from the fixation point at the time of exposure and had allowed the test word to be projected to the left hemisphere. Also, the stimuli so named were rerun and intermixed in the series, yielding no consistent above-chance performance. With these rare exceptions, it was clear from the verbal responses that the left hemisphere was only guessing and that knowledge of the correct answer had been confined to the right hemisphere.

Spelling

Tests were run to find out to what degree the right hemisphere might have the ability to order and arrange individual letters into words. Alphabet letters about 4 inches high, cut from heavy cardboard, were presented out of vision to the left hand for manual palpation and arrangement. Thus the patients had only to feel and recognize the individual letters and then place them in correct spatial order from left to right. Case II failed to perform convincingly, but the significance of this is questionable in view of the left-handed hypoesthesia. Only Case III was able to spell consistently with the subordinate hemisphere, as indicated in results like the following: The subject was told to spell a word like "dog," after which the examiner placed the appropriate three letters, one at a time in random order, into the subject's left hand for placement on the table. Very simple familiar words, like "how," "what," "pie," and "hat," were spelled correctly under these conditions, but only slowly and with considerable effort. When an occasional mistake was made in letter order, the examiner would suggest that the subject check the word, and usually the error was found and corrected on the first check. During this particular test, wherein the left hemisphere also heard, the subject would often talk in a confabulatory way. Thus, while holding the "O" for "dog" in his left hand, the subject would say, "That's the 'D'." Nevertheless, the left hand would continue to spell correctly, demonstrating the ability of the minor hemisphere to maintain its own reasoning, will, and intent in the presence of competitive ideas and other distracting influences from the major hemisphere.

In further tests, a group of three or four letters was presented, out of vision, to the left hand, and the subjects were instructed to "spell a word." The word to be spelled was not stated, and it remained for the right hemisphere to recognize the individual letters and to arrange them into meaningful order. Case III again proved able to do this, and spelled such words as "cup," "not," "cake," "love," and "what."

Calculation

With stimuli presented tactually to the minor hemisphere through the left hand, Cases II and III demonstrated a limited ability to add correctly the numbers 1 or 2, to numbers under 10. They were unable, however, to subtract or multiply at this level. In this test, a set of one to four wooden pegs (2.5 x 0.8 cm) implanted upright in 2-inch wooden blocks was presented to the patients left hand, out of view, and in random order. Initially, it was shown that the patients, upon command, could readily pick out blocks 1, 2, or 3, etc. With a card with printed numbers from 1 to 8 placed in open view in front of the patients, two blocks were serially presented to the left hand and the patients were required to point with the left hand to the number representing the sum. They usually succeeded with the numbers under 5, but were unable to subtract the number of pegs in one block from those in another, or to double or triple the number of pegs. In a more recent follow-up study, Sperry (1968a) estimated the ability to calculate to be at a higher level than described in the foregoing.

All of the above tasks, of course, were performed easily with the other hand. In addition, much more complicated problems and general experience with the use of mathematics, changing money, estimating food quantities, and so forth, all made it questionable that calculations carried out with the major hemisphere were at all impaired. Case III had some difficulty during the fourth and fifth months after surgery in carrying out written mathematical calculation. This proved to be a problem not so much in the ability to calculate per se, but in taking care to scan far enough to the left so that all numbers fell in the right half field.

SUMMARY

Some of the main points that emerge in the foregoing regarding the cerebral organization of language and the cerebral disconnection syndrome generally, may be summarized briefly as follows. Information perceived exclusively or generated exclusively in the minor (right) hemisphere could be communicated neither in speech nor in writing; it had to be expressed entirely through nonverbal responses. By contrast, there was no noticeable impairment of speech and writing with reference to information processed in the major (left) hemisphere. Linguistic expression seemed, thus, to be organized almost exclusively in the left hemisphere. The possibility that a few simple emotional, tonal, or extremely familiar words might be expressed through the minor hemisphere in these cases, however, cannot be completely ruled out from the present data.

In contrast to the highly lateralized organization of verbal expression, the comprehension of language, both spoken and written, was found to be represented in the minor as well as in the major hemisphere. Present evidence indicates that the minor hemisphere is less proficient than the major in this respect. Performances with the right hemisphere involving word and object association, sorting, retrieval, and related tasks showed evidence of ideation, emotion, mental concentration, and other high-order mental capacities.

The observed ability to write with the left hand legible and meaningful material, though with rather poor penmanship, can be explained in terms of the bilateral motor control of both hands from the major hemisphere. Therefore, it is not a contradiction of the above conclusion that writing is organized only in the major hemisphere. The bilaterality in motor control applies to a lesser degree to the control of the right hand from the minor hemisphere. This latter combination is clearly inferior to the above, in part because the dominant hemisphere tends to interfere more by imposing its own control on the right hand.

The foregoing applies also to the drawing of simple objects and geometric shapes perceived either visually or stereognostically. After presentation to the major hemisphere either hand could draw the object, but the performance was clearly superior with the right hand. Following such presentation to the minor right hemisphere, the left hand drew moderately recognizable reproductions. Drawing with the right, however, was highly erratic under these conditions and was commonly disrupted by interfering functions in the major hemisphere.

The evidence that the disconnected minor hemisphere perceives and comprehends both the written and spoken word contrasts with previous reports of "word blindness" and "word deafness" following callosal lesions (Geschwind, 1965a, b). Since the present two patients also appeared alexic and "word blind" in tests that involved verbal communication, one wonders if the application of appropriate nonverbal testing methods might not have demonstrated the presence of comprehension in the minor hemisphere in the earlier studies as well. Also the earlier cases of word blindness and deafness involved extensive cortical lesions in the dominant hemisphere. It becomes increasingly evident that the functional capacity of a unilateral cortical area with its contralateral counterpart intact may appear to be quite different from that seen in the presence of contralateral lesions. Allowing for considerable individual variation in the cerebral organization of language, the general picture as outlined in the present cases could well prove to be more typical than exceptional so far as we can tell from the evidence now available.

Many of the studies reported in this chapter point out some of the ways the brain-bisected primate is able to maintain a facade of perceptual unity despite the complete disconnection of the cerebral commissures. While the profound incapacity of information transfer between the two half-brains after mid-line commissure surgery remains, "jumping the split" can be accomplished through some of the neural mechanisms and behavioral strategies outlined above such as: eye divergence, cooperative strategies, emotional cross-cuing, ipsilateral somatosensory representation, and target information cross over.

To some extent, cross-cuing mechanisms are but a sample of the many methods the neurologic patient has available to cheat, as it were, on any of a number of particular clinical examinations. The old problem of administering proper examinations to the endlessly clever primate—to be receiving data relevant to the examiner's question—is seen in new and varied forms in cases of brain bisection. Indeed, many of the cuing systems described here may be operative in traditional cases of brain lesion. Any substantial cortical lesion in associative cortex will produce a partial split-brain because of the associated callosal degeneration. The disconnection effects that could conceivably be unearthed in such cases might well be overlooked because of the patient's ability to switch to a cross-cuing mechanism thereby leaving the real neurologic state confounded.

In somatosensory or motor-lesion cases, the human clinical patient might not reveal the extent of his deficit. For example, with a right parietal lesion, complete stereognostic recognition for the left hand might in reality be lost. Yet, in tests it appears the patient can describe many of the familiar objects presented to him for examination. Here, as in the split, ipsilateral cuing systems relaying only quantitative information about the stimulus might be sufficiently informative to cue the left speech hemisphere into a correct response. In some cases this would lead to a conclusion the right-hemisphere lesion might not have been extensive enough or that secondary somatosensory areas exist in the right hemisphere which are able to handle the task under consideration. These interpretations, of course, would be far afield if this particular patient was using a self-cuing strategy of the type described.

7

Cerebral Dominance and Lateral Specialization

The task of locating and defining where in the human brain certain specialized functions of higher mental activity reside is of great interest, not only because an analog does not exist in subhuman primates, but also because it raises serious questions for those trying to understand the developmental logic of cerebral organization. With each passing year, new data are brought out demonstrating that there is more of this or that aspect of mental life on the right than on the left, or more on the left than on the right (Milner, 1962). This distribution of duties in the cerebrum in what appears to be a highly ordered fashion we assume to be the product of some as yet undetermined neural logic. Approaching an understanding of this phenomenon is the aim of this chapter, and the task taken will be to examine the problem in the light of a variety of split-brain data and prejudices. First, some of the specialized functions of the left and the right hemisphere unearthed in tests of the brain-bisected patients will be reviewed, and will be contrasted with what some believe to be the functional state of each hemisphere in the young child. These psychologic considerations will then be integrated with the studies on hemisphere-hand relations in both split-brain monkeys and man, and a novel interpretation of the developing cerebrum, which suggests that the normal neonate is born, for all practical purposes, with a split-brain. If the latter proposition proves to be halfway reasonable, the neonate is subject to a certain class of phenomena that might assist the understanding of the development of lateralized language and speech.

What can an adult disconnected right hemisphere do? We have already shown in Chapter 6 that it is essentially identical in function and ability to the left hemisphere on such tasks as the following: Simple and choice reaction times are the same; intermodal transfer from vision to touch and touch to vision is intact and for familiar objects appears as efficient on the right as on the left; likewise, auditory-tactual and auditory-visual matches are realized on the right as well as on the left. The ability to emote to provocative stimuli is intact and present in the right hemisphere as well as the left hemisphere. The right hemisphere can learn any of a number of visual and tactual problems with the same rapidity as the left hemisphere. In short-term-memory experiments, the right hemisphere is found to be as good (or bad) as the left. The ability to control the contralateral motor system is intact, and the right hemisphere is as good in controlling the left half of the body as the left hemisphere is good in controlling the right. Stereognostic recognition for the left hand is present and intact in the right hemisphere, and vice versa; and so the list goes.

The major differences between the right and left hemispheres are seen in the analysis of language and speech systems. The left hemisphere is of course capable of speech, whereas the adult right hemisphere is predictably incapable. Information presented to the left hemisphere is normally handled, but identical stimulation of the right yields no response.

More interestingly, studies on language comprehension again show the left hemisphere undisturbed by the operation, with no interruption in the linguistic system observable. But, what about the right hemisphere? Again, as shown in Chapter 6, it is found that the right hemisphere understands *some* language. In brief, the right hemisphere can handle concrete nouns. Flash the word "pencil" to the right hemisphere, with a request to retrieve the corresponding object from a series with the left hand, and the patient experiences no difficulty. At the same time, this type of test procedure reveals that the right hemisphere can in no way respond to verbs, that is, simple printed-out commands. Flash the commands "laugh," "smile," "tap," "hit," and so on, to the left hemisphere, and there is no problem. But flash these requests to the right hemisphere, and the patient fails to make a response. The best language-rich patients are even unable to point to a picture that best portrays the action. Also, the right hemisphere can recognize affirmative and negative constructions, but is not able to recognize active-passive constructions, or future constructions, or pluralizations, and the like. In general, then, the overall language capacity of the right hemisphere is limited, and of a particular kind.

When the data are juxtaposed with observations made on the brain-lesioned young child (which in essence points up that the right hemisphere as well as the left possesses a great deal of language [Basser, 1962]), one becomes aware of a striking contrast. It seems clear that up to a certain level of development, each hemisphere processes and records some linguistic information. The data further suggest that the capacity, at a minimum, is advanced to handle such things as nouns, verbs, and the like. In the adult disconnected right hemisphere, however, we fail to unearth even these miniature linguistic systems. What happened? Where does the language competence present in the young child's right hemisphere go?

Further, on this same general point, some recent results of ours indicate that the normal adult does not rely on the right hemisphere for handling a simple language analysis. Using an adaptation of Posner's physical identity-name-identity test (Posner and Mitchell, 1967), three conditions were run on six normal subjects. The basic test is to respond as fast as possible to whether two letters, say AA, are the same or different from, say, AB. The second phase is to see how much longer it takes to label the same name, say Aa, but not Ab. That is, in the second test, the subject must *not* respond to physical identity, but rather to whether the letters have the same name. Posner found that it takes about 71 msec longer for name identity. Our test was to see if it made a difference which hemisphere saw the test stimulus. The idea here is that if the right hemisphere does not have extensive language function normally, it ought to take longer to respond because the information would have to first relayed over to the left hemisphere for analysis. Differences, however, should not show up in the physical identity test, which requires no language analysis. Our preliminary results confirmed this view. When the test is presented in the right visual field, that is the left hemisphere, the name-identity test can be done significantly faster than when the stimuli are presented to the right hemisphere. However, both hemispheres respond alike in rate to the physical-identity test. In brief, then, the findings support the view that the adult right hemisphere carries out very little language activity in the normal state. We shall try to make sense of this observation later.

A second consideration for the hypothesis is to examine what is occurring in the underlying neurologic organization of cortical development. More specifically, the aim will be to describe the functional development of the large interhemispheric commissure in man, the corpus callosum. The point will be that there is at least suggestive evidence that the human neonate is a split-brain for a good period of time, and is thus subject to a special class of phenomena that is not apparent in the non-split-brain.

Contrary to several textbook descriptions of the issue, recent observations (Hewitt, 1962) on the developing corpus callosum are of interest. In brief, his results indicate that the interhemispheric structure is not functional at birth, and that great parts of it remain undeveloped during early life. He finds "at birth the callosum is incompletely established and only bears a superficial resemblance to the adult form. It is relatively narrow in depth or thickness. Subsequent additions to the commissure would not be unexpected if its growth parallels that of the cortex . . . i.e., it builds up as different areas of the cortex mature." In general, then, the developmental course coincides with the development of the cortex, with the more primary sensory areas becoming functionally active first, and the more associative areas last.

What statements of this kind mean in terms of neural tissue is still not known. The general scheme, however, is entirely consistent with the views of Langworthy (1933) that tracts in the nervous system become myelinated at the time when they become functional. Add to this the exhaustive studies of Conel (1941, 1959) on the development of the human cortex, and we find that myelination and overall development are an ongoing process in most active fashion during the first two years of life, and continue in a less vigorous manner up to puberty. In summary, then, the ordering of the developing cerebrum is of such a nature that it allows our hypothesis that the young infant is to some extent a "split-brain." This would suggest that interhemispheric communication is slight at birth, and increases with age, with good communication seen for all conditions starting around the ages of two to three.

Add to this the studies on the split-brain that deal with the effects on learning of controlled hand use. Split-brain monkeys, when learning a visual pattern discrimination with both eyes open, and in full view of the stimulus, but limited in response to using only one hand, usually lay down engrams in only one hemisphere (Trevarthen, 1962; Gazzaniga, 1963). That is, even though the whole organism looks as though it now "knows" the problem, separate testing of each eye after the animal has reached criterion reveals that only one eye-hemisphere knows the problem. Furthermore, it is usually the contralateral eye to the responding hand. If the right hand is used in response, it is the left hemisphere which can perform the task when tested singly; if the left hand is used in response, it is the right hemisphere which knows the problem.

Conversely, when free-hand choice is allowed, but only one eye is exposed to the stimulus, a split-brain monkey tends to perform with the contralateral hand. There is, then, a clear link between eye and hand, and intrahemispheric pairs are dominant.

These same relations have also been seen in the tests with split-brain patients, as described in Chapter 6. Here, patients are flashed two different stimuli, one in the left visual field, and therefore exclusively projected to the right hemisphere, and one in the right visual field, and therefore projected to only the left hemisphere. If the subject is asked to point with the left hand to the stimuli seen in the flash, the response will be to the figure projected to the right hemisphere. If the subject is asked to point with the right hand, the subject will point to the flash projected to the left hemisphere. This has been observed repeatedly over the several years of testing of these patients.

The foregoing observations hopefully tie together and allow for a hypothesis about some of the factors active in the development of cerebral dominance and lateral specialization. The idea is that the neonate is viewed as an extremely exploratory creature, with a split, or partially split, brain. Between one and two years of age, the prediction would be that as the child manipulates toys, food, and a variety of other objects, with a slightly greater frequency with his right than his left hand, engram formation and the central distribution of learned material would be centered in the left hemisphere. The experimental studies on the monkey would suggest this. As mentioned above, learning which takes place during right-hand exploration is centered in the left hemisphere; learning taking place during left-hand activity would be processed in the right hemisphere. It is herein suggested it would mean the same for the young child. When the child was set to explore with the right hand, visual, auditory, or tactual engrams would be established in the left hemisphere. The same would be true for a left hand set with the engrams being laid down on the right. Since it is predicted that more explorations would be with the right hand, however, the left hemisphere would quickly develop a lead. Consequently, since the left hemisphere would soon know more, it would also ask more questions of its environment, which in turn would be read out as more and more right-hand activity. Hand use reinforces hemisphere use, and quickly enough, hemisphere competence reinforces hand use, with the result that the two systems in a circular fashion mutually reinforce each other.

Consistent with this view is the prediction that the right hemisphere in the young child would develop a language system separately and of its own. It is functionally disconnected from the left according to the hypothesis, and so would establish its own engrams when a child was set to use the left hand. This means, however, that while the right did possess some language, it would not be as proficient as the left at any stage in development, and it would become less and less so as development took place. This fits the neurological data. Left-hemisphere lesions in the young child do not cause a total disruption in language capacity, as they do in adults, which indicates that the right hemisphere has separately developed some language competence.

The final step in this notion would be to consider what occurs when the corpus callosum becomes functionally hooked up in the adult form, at around the age of two. The neurologic observations, starting at this point in development, indicate that left-hemisphere lesions become more and more disruptive with respect to language, hereby indicating that these processes are more and more entrenched in the left hemisphere. In other words, dominance is waxing, and information duplication is waning. Could it be that these phenomena are related?

Imagine the situation where two separate brains are viewing the world. Whichever one happens to be attentive at a particular moment will establish engrams for the situation at hand. As the brains become more communicative with each other, that is, as the corpus callosum hooks up to the point where everything experienced by one hemisphere is instantly communicated to the other, a different logic would emerge for the recording and processing of memory. The lead hemisphere, the dominant left, would be attending to external information and, while receiving and processing it, would be holding the other disengaged. Thus, duplication of engrams and learning in general would be less frequent, with the net result that the left hemisphere would become more and more dominant. The information on the right would be used less frequently, and over a period of time during development, would perhaps be lost, or erased, or even functionally suppressed.

The scheme would explain the contrast seen between the adult's and child's right hemisphere mentioned earlier. In summary, the view is that some evidence exists that the young child has a partially split-brain. It would therefore be subject to a certain class of phenomena which, in the main, would encourage or enhance lateral development of language.

8

Early Versus Late Lesions— More Apparent than Real

Few phenomena in neuropsychology have more important implications for a general theory of brain function than the one presently under discussion. The differential effects of early versus late lesions in the performance of motor, sensory, and a wide variety of behavioral tasks stands out as a true enigma. One of the emerging concepts of this work, functional sparing, is so bold in its attack on nativism that the issue must be dealt with head-on. Either the neurocircuit design of the neonate is completely established by informational systems revealed through hereditary mechanisms, or it isn't; either the developing zygote programs the organizational logic of the frontal, temporal, parietal, and visual lobes, or it doesn't; either the primary features of the brain are built-in or are added with experience.

To be sure, the point is not that it is either nature or nurture, a dichotomy that surfaced in a time when there wasn't much else to talk about in the behavior-related sciences. The concept that an interaction between the environment and the organismic hardware produces the final behavior product is fine, but it should not be forgotten that this view does not negate the more basic point that the primary neurocircuits and organizations are laid down according to a specific set of instructions. Whether the initial capacity of the system is maximized depends upon environmental contingencies.

The objective of the present chapter is to maintain that early-late data do not really speak to the issue of whether behavioral nerve nets are prewired. The argument will be that sparing, in the sense implied by this work, is not a reality. In brief, the data from early versus late brain-bisection studies suggest that early-lesioned organisms, when tested as adults, perform a task by alternate mechanisms, not relocated mechanisms, as a result of early lesions. The callosal agenesis case seems to appear integrated across the split, not because of newly formed aberrant neurological pathways, but perhaps because the patients are enormously clever at developing behavioral strategies to deal with their physical incapacities. Indeed, it will be argued that when these cross-cuing strategies are eliminated or not allowed as part of the test sequence, the agenesis case shows many of the same kind of incapacities as seen in the surgically sectioned adult. The following then, is a case report of a patient first examined by me some years ago.

The patient was first studied at California Institute of Technology in December of 1961. His mother, a registered nurse, had spotted an item in a newspaper concerning the effects of callosal surgery in the monkey, and had written to ask whether any new work might contribute to the understanding of her son's problem.

Examination of the patient's medical record revealed the following: He was first seen at the age of 11 years, in December, 1952, at which time diagnostic studies were made including pneumoencephalograph, which definitely established agenesis of the corpus callosum, as well as cortical atrophy and dilated lateral ventricles. EEGs were made which showed subcortical encephalopathy, projected mainly to the right temporal and right occipital areas. Psychological testing revealed the I.Q. in the dull-to-normal range, and that he had very poor eye-hand coordination. This latter condition improved throughout the years. His nursery-school reports revealed him to be a corrigible and easy-going lad, with language facility ahead of his years, but curiously, with poor space perception. It was reported that at the age of five he would step over half-inch objects with a 12-to14-inch clearance.

While frustratingly lazy, the boy was very happy and jolly. When talking with the examiner alone, he pointed out that his sister wanted to be a doctor. He then quickly added, with a smile, that he didn't think she would make it because she gets failing marks in school. He seemed to lack depth perception: when walking down the corridor, he would put his hands out in front of him when approaching a door. The gesture seemed to indicate that he didn't see the door at all, unless searching for it.

The patient was reexamined seven months later, and again was found to be happy and affable. He remained a difficult person to test, and would constantly try to cheat, or, more simply, did not care what sort of response he made. At this time, his parents described his handedness history. According to them, he wrote with his right hand, and also ate with his right hand. With his left hand he threw baseballs and performed similar tasks. The parents voluntarily said, "He seems to do more aggressive things with his left hand."

The patient was first examined over a three-day period. In general, his personality, temperament, and overall affect appeared healthy and buoyant. Contrary to the majority view in the literature, he did not appear subnormal or dull.

In our psychologic and neurologic testing of the patient, we used those procedures established and developed for the testing of our adult brain-bisection patients, as described in Chapter 6. Using this general orientation, it is possible to question whether visual information projected to one hemisphere transfers or can get together with visual information projected to the other. The same is also true for somatosensory stimulation.

In general, all neurologic and psychologic testing revealed a remarkable ability to cross-integrate information presented in one hemisphere with information presented to the other. Visual stimuli, for example, when flashed to the left hemisphere could be normally named and described, but information flashed exclusively to the right hemisphere could also be named and described. This finding, of course, stands in marked contrast to the data collected on the brain-bisected adults, where it was clearly seen that information projected to the left hemisphere could be named and normally described, but information projected to the right could not.

In tests of stereognosis, the agenesis case could easily verbally describe objects placed in either hand out of view. In our brain-bisected adult, stereognostic recognition was possible only for objects held in the right hand. Objects held in the left hand of our brain-bisected adults could be manipulated correctly, but because the critical tactile information was exclusively projected to the right hemisphere, the patient could not verbally describe the palpated objects.

There are a number of possible explanations for these disparate findings. One obvious hypothesis is, of course, that there are interhemispheric commissures remaining, which have taken on new and high level function, and that these systems are now capable of handling the kind of interhemispheric information transmission that is necessary to perform these tasks. It is, for example, the case that callosal agenesis patients have a rather well-developed anterior commissure. Some argue that this may be the neural path for the rerouting of high-level information-transmission duties.

It strikes me that this kind of neurologizing is nothing but handwaving, for serious consideration of the implications of the foregoing lead one to conclude that the whole circuit diagram of the developing neocortex can, with a little nudging, be totally reorganized.

An alternative view would be that there is no serious cross-integration of information between the two hemispheres, even in the agenesis case. The notion that I would like to propose moves from the axiom that in cases of callosal agenesis, both hemispheres have developed language and speech systems (a similar view has recently been advanced by Sperry (1968a). (There is one known, documented exception to this view, worked out by Milner [personal communication]. She had a case tested with unilateral injections of amytol, which showed a speech center on one side only.) Nonetheless, it is the view that when the patient is able to describe objects held in the left hand, it is not because the stereognostic information has been relayed to the right hemisphere and then over to the left speech hemisphere, but rather because the right hemisphere is also able to talk. Likewise, when he is able to describe stimuli presented in the left visual field, it is not because the left speech hemisphere is interpreting information coming through the anterior commissure or whatever, but again because the right hemisphere has its own speech mechanism and can describe the object directly. With this basic mechanism existing in the agenesis case, it is easy, indeed, to imagine all the ways one hemisphere could cross-cue the other as to what is going on. If, for example, the phrase "ham and eggs" is flashed, such that half falls into one visual field and half falls into the other, and the patient is asked what he saw, he says with no uncertainty, "Ham and eggs." As soon as the right hemisphere says "ham," the left hemisphere not only hears that, but supplies the eggs, so that quick enough, both hemispheres know the full content of the message. Or more simply, when a visual stimulus, say the word "egg," is flashed into the left field, the right hemisphere straightaway identifies the stimulus. No cross-integration whatsoever is needed here.

The hypothesis raises two questions. First, if the agenesis case is really the ideal split—that is, a patient with two completely separate language and speech systems—why are they not more often in conflict? The answer, here, would be that the developing system is hopelessly tied together. What one brain sees is also seen by the other. What the environmental contingencies are that effect some particular kind of emotion will also be experienced by the other simultaneously, and so on.

The second question is, if cross-cuing strategies are eliminated, does the agenesis case look more like the adult surgically split patient? The data suggest that this is the case. In the one-test run, where no verbal report was made concerning input into one hemisphere, thereby leaving the other in the dark save for possible neurological mechanisms, the opposite hemisphere was unable to act appropriately. The test was as follows:

The subject's hand was placed under a partition, and out of view. The test first required the patient to localize, with the thumb of one hand, a point lightly stimulated on that hand. Thus, over a series of trials, several points on each finger were stimulated.

In the second phase of testing, the patient was required to locate the corresponding point of stimulation on the opposite hand. If, for example, the patient was stimulated on the right index finger, the test would be to find the left index finger with the left thumb.

In previous testing of the brain-bisected adults, as reported in Chapter 6, it has been unequivocally shown that this test could be carried out so long as stimulus and response were kept to the same side. As long as the right thumb was responding to stimulation of points on the right hand, there was no difficulty; and likewise, for the left hand responding to left hand stimulation.

Correct performance broke down in the brain-bisected patients, however, when cross-integration of information was required. Thus, the left thumb was unable to find a corresponding point of stimulation on the right hand. The same was true the other way around. These findings have held up and endured through six years of testing on the brain-bisected patients.

In testing the one agenesis case, we obtained the same results.

The patient was accurate when stimulus and response were kept to the same side. The left thumb could find left hand points and the right thumb could find right hand points. The left thumb, however, was unable to point to the corresponding area stimulated on the right side, and vice versa.

Thus, when cross-cuing is eliminated—that is, when one hemisphere is not allowed to tell the answer to the other side—the split effect is seen. The prediction would be that if callosal agenesis cases were tested with this problem in mind, more disconnection phenomena would be observed. Or, with respect to Milner's case, straightforward split-brain tests ought to reveal at least some of these striking symptoms. It is worthwhile noting, as an aside, that these cross-cuing strategies can become extremely sophisticated, and unless one is attuned to this mechanism, one can be seriously misled as to the meaning of a particular piece of behavior. This is constantly seen when the novice tries his hand at examining commissure-lesioned patients, and great precaution must be executed.

The foregoing would predict that agenesis in animals ought to reveal a syndrome more akin to the surgical cases. In a recent elegant experiment by Yamagouchi and Myers (1969) newborn monkeys underwent commissurotomy in the first week of life. In subsequent testing at a later date transfer tests on brightness, color, and pattern discrimination found the early-lesioned monkeys displaying the same dramatic loss of integration routinely seen in adult surgically split animals! Of course, essential differences conceivably could exist between agenesis and neonatal surgical preparations, and might negate these findings.

More generally, the point of the foregoing argument is that early lesions in the corpus callosum do not result in a fundamental reorganization of the hemispheric commissure data-exchange system. It is conceivable that the remaining systems take on an increased load, but it would be viewed more as a quantitative increase in activity, than as a qualitative one.

9

An Overview
and New Directions

A curious aspect of split-brain research is the oblique way it speaks to any particular theory of brain function. The startling phenomenon itself offers little insight into the mysteries of mind and brain in terms of illuminating real neural mechanisms. In some sense, it mischievously doubles the magnitude of the problem and raises more questions than it answers. Certainly there are few, if any, propositions in neurobiology that would be rejected or accepted on the basis of the original split-brain experiments.

A great deal of the split-brain enterprise involves using the method as a technique to study some of the traditional problems outstanding in neuropsychology. It is in a way the fall-out that raises so many questions and offers so many new angles on a wide variety of issues. The studies do not offer up a unified view of brain function; nor can they be summarized in terms of an overall theory, for the bulk of the studies quite clearly are looking at a number of separate and isolated ideas about brain mechanisms, which to this day remain largely unstructured and lack a clear interrelation.

Most of the specific ideas and integrations possible from the many studies reviewed have been spelled out in the preceding chapters. As a final effort, the following discussion presents some overviews on a number of problems in brain function and then moves on to outline some possibilities for new directions in split-brain research.

Right Hemisphere Function

Clinical studies of unilateral brain injury, as well as the split-brain studies described in Chapter 6, enumerate a number of mental attributes present in the minor right hemisphere of man. The cerebral taxonomy of mental life is of enormous interest but still leaves unanswered the general question of what the predominant function is of one entire half of the human cerebrum. The meager list of its assets unearthed to date hardly appears adequate to explain its role in light of the amount of neural tissue involved.

A persistent idea arising from split-brain studies is that the right hemisphere's most important function is to allow for "echo time" in the processing of incoming information. The results of Day's experiment, mentioned in Chapter 6 (p. 89), can be interpreted in this light. The poor performance of patients with complete callosal transection on temporal-order recall tests, as the time between sounds increases, serves as a possible striking example of this notion. The findings have all the appearances of a basic short-term memory deficit—a difficulty of retrieving serially presented information—by putting on hold Bit A while Bit B is being outputted. The notion of a poor reverberatory circuit system or echo-time system might also explain why in the visual tests of short term memory, described in Chapter 6, the split-brain patients were much poorer than normal patients within a given hemisphere.

Consistent with the view is the suggestion by MacKay (1967, personal communication) that the right hemisphere might serve to qualify statements made by the left. The frequency of saying "but" or "however" might then be reduced in split-brain subjects. The idea here is that the right hemisphere would be "thinking" of the qualifications of the ongoing statements by listening to the left hemisphere and then serving notice on the left hemisphere when to qualify or modify the content of a particular declaration. Recently, Hall et al. (1968) reported that patients with right cerebral lesions did not qualify statements made, to the extent observed in patients with left cerebral lesions. Likewise, the fascinating studies of Doty (1969) on what he termed "butterflies in the brain" might be relevant here. In awake monkeys implanted with electrodes in visual cortex, stimulation elicited a general orientation response coupled with reaching movements of the contralateral hand to a particular point in space followed by what appeared to be a grasping movement for an object. Subsequently, at the cessation of stimulation, the animals looked dismayed when upon opening their hands they discovered they had not "caught" the object. What is of particular interest here is that only split-brain animals responded in this fashion! Normal animals would not respond to similar, unilateral stimulation of the visual cortex, as if the opposite side checked or qualified the intentions of the stimulated hemisphere. Could it be that this all fits together?

If one places these notions in the more general context of the need for "echo time" I think the idea becomes helpful. The matter could be viewed in terms of the right hemisphere allowing for the necessary reverberation time thereby enabling the system to check and cross-check the proposition and subsequently possibly to initiate qualifying remarks. This removes the necessity of having the right hemisphere responsible for the "but" or "however" function per se, and puts the idea into the framework of what might be called the need for "processing space." Certainly the exchange of information and the subroutines active and called upon during short-term memory would require an enormous network and information-exchange system. Separating or destroying the processing system usually active in assisting the propositional system, namely the right hemisphere, would indeed have the effects observed in the foregoing studies.

Split-Brain and Conscious Experience

One of the persistent inferences made from split-brain studies is that midsagittal sectioning of the cerebral commissures produces a state of mental duplicity; that two separate conscious spheres coexist within one cranium. Without taking on the difficult task of defining what consciousness is or is not, the approach has been simply to spell out what each hemisphere of the split-brain animal can or cannot do, separately and independently. In man, the qualitative aspects of right and left cerebral function have been analyzed with the score for the presence or absence of a variety of functions for each half-brain recorded. While this is acceptable on an operational basis, it does beg the question.

The assertion of the existence of double consciousness (Sperry, 1964a, 1964b, 1966, 1968b; Gazzaniga, 1967b) has been contested by Eccles (1965). In general, the arguments on both sides deal with judgments on the amount of data available to make the inference. MacKay (1966), on the other hand, who has made some specific suggestions as to the mechanical basis of consciousness, specifically contends that the studies to date have not examined the critical dimension, namely the presence or absence of separate priority-determining systems for each hemisphere. If this aspect of the information system is common to both hemispheres then he is not prepared to dub each side as separate, conscious units. This is an important point.

Clearly, there are certain aspects of brain and humoral activity not split in these patients. Both left and right neural systems bathe in the same humoral pools and both are linked in electrophysiologic response to a variety of stimuli. The question becomes how many normative physiologic mechanisms are common to both hemispheres. MacKay thinks this is crucial, for he contends that this is the essential correlate of consciousness—what he calls the "meta-organizing system," the system that sets the goals, the priorities, the rank order of objectives for an organism.

The only split-brain experiment that speaks to this issue is an unpublished study of mine carried out on monkeys several years ago. Split-brain monkeys, wearing goggles, were allowed to view a plate of red and green grapes with one eye. They freely ate an assortment of both kinds. Subsequently, the opposite eye alone viewed a different tray of green grapes flavored with quinine, and untreated red grapes. After only one or two trials the green grapes were avoided and only the red grapes were retrieved for eating. When the first eye was retested, would it now be that a different value for green grapes had been assigned to them and they would now be avoided? Apparently not, for without hestitation both kinds were picked up with equal frequency. One would think if the goal-directing system were common to both hemispheres, the reordering of values that took place in the second hemisphere would be known to the opposite hemisphere.

The problem with the experiment, of course, is that the monkeys could have been doing the task on a conditional basis. That is, the animal might "decide," when using the right eye, that the grapes were all acceptable, but when using the left eye, only the red ones were acceptable. If this had been the strategy, then split or not the experiment did not address the issue under investigation. This general problem once understood, intrudes on any number of designs that one might offer in order to test the proposition. As a result, the question of the extent of the duplication of conscious mechanisms by midsaggital section of the cerebral commissures, I think, remains open.

Derepression of Prewired Circuits

A common and frustrating aspect of brain-lesion work is the fact that lost function returns with time. Deficits of one kind or another seen in the first weeks or months after surgery disappear eventually. This is not always the case, of course, for there are instances of persistent deficits such as the effects of infratemporal lesions on visual learning. Nonetheless, the phenomenon is encountered frequently, with several cases in split-brain research being of particular interest.

The partial commissure section studies reported in Chapter 5 are relevant. In studies on the monkey, sectioning the splenium only momentarily stops interhemispheric transfer of visual learning in the chiasm-sectioned monkey. After the animal has been trained on a few problems, transfer reappears only to be stopped by additionally sectioning the anterior commissure.

In somatosensory testing of the human, one gains the clear impression of an increase in functional capacity in ipsilateral systems with time. While most of the improvement is probably a function of discovering psychologic strategies as described in Chapter 3, some room must be left open for the possibility that latent pathways were activated.

On the motor side, brain-bisection studies demonstrate that animals with what are regarded as major motor and sensory systems separated from one another remain capable of performing integrated activities. While the data presented in Chapter 4 argue strongly for cross-cuing systems to explain many of the studies reported to date, the possibility remains that ipsilateral cortical spinal systems are activated to handle the deficits impressed by the surgery.

Lastly, of course, the dramatic differences seen in cases of callosal agenesis versus surgical cases raise a series of questions about the possibility of multiple subcallosal pathways being involved in interhemispheric synthesis of information. The argument presented in Chapter 8 centers on the notion that most of the findings can be explained away by cross-cuing strategies. Still, the distinct possibility remains that some, if not all, synthesis takes place through neurological channels.

All such data suggest a phenomenon of brain surgery that might be called the derepression of prewired circuits. Implicit in the notion, of course, is that reorganization of the subcircuits themselves does not take place. Rather, the switching mechanism, or the system choosing which subroutine to use, hunts further into its library of response repertoires to find a possible program that would work under a particular set of conditions. This, of course, need not be a program entirely specific for those sets of conditions, but merely one encompassing those conditions.

Possible Rehabilitory Strategies for Mental Development in Brain-Damaged Children

Throughout most of the split-brain research, the idea of efficient intrahemispheric communication being dominant over behavior tasks requiring interhemispheric systems is most common. Keeping activities requiring sensory-motor interaction confined to one hemisphere greatly enhances performance, as described in Chapters 3 and 4. With hemisphere disconnection, difficulties arise, as noted throughout the book in a number of contexts. The problem is most clearly seen in surgical section cases where the hemispheres are cleanly and completely separated at the cortical level. Hemisphere disconnection can also result, of course, from the degeneration of the callosal fibers normally innervating a region of extirpated or damaged cortex. Such lesions produce a partial commissurotomy, much like those produced surgically as described in Chapter 5, and they also result in the same behavioral characteristics. For example, a unilateral lesion in the second somatosensory area of the cat prevents the routine interhemispheric transfer of tactile learning that is seen in the normal cat (Teitlebaum et al., 1968). Disconnection effects have also frequently been seen in humans with brain damage (Geschwind and Kaplan, 1962). Similar interpretations have been suggested for still other related phenomena occurring in brain damaged man (Gazzaniga et al., 1962). Rather frequent bilateral deficits occur following left unilateral cerebral lesions. This might well be attributed in part to interruption of sensory material due to hemisphere disconnection resulting from the brain damage, thereby creating a situation where information arriving in the right hemisphere would remain isolated there instead of being normally transmitted to the left half-brain for language and speech interpretation and response.

This kind of data suggests that if one looks at the brain not as a whole but as two equal halves that could incur partial or total disconnection due to a brain lesion, alternative procedures for rehabilitating and training of children are generated that run contrary to some present notions including the idea that a natural interrelation between eye and hand dominance exists in visual-motor learning. The training and rehabilitation procedure based on these theories, as well as others, may prove to be disappointing to brain-damaged children especially when hope for real rehabilitation is alive. The reason for this is that under certain conditions of eye and hand training imposed on the child by the therapist, sensory-sensory, or sensory-motor integration would be implicitly required across a disconnected or partially disconnected brain, and it is now known that such integration is not possible or at best is difficult.

Possible alternative methods generated out of the studies presented herein would argue for encouraging sensory-motor activities to be channeled through the same hemisphere. Instead, for example, of encouraging visual exposure in the unilaterally brain-injured child through the dominant eye in combination with the ipsilateral hand, the rationale would be to encourage exposing visual material in the visual half-field directly, intrahemispherically related to the responding hand. Assuming the responding hand received its major motor control from the undamaged hemisphere, the method would potentiate the most efficient sensory-motor system available in the damaged brain in addition to encouraging the attentional processes critical to learning to be centered in that hemisphere. If the working hemisphere did not happen to be dominant for speech, this activity would not necessarily impair synthesis of the visual-motor activity with the speech mechanisms on the dominant side, for interhemispheric pathways would still be available for interhemispheric communication by virtue of the fact that relevant commissural systems would remain intact.

Variations of this general suggestion are abundant, and each neurologic problem would argue for its own particular solution. Whether or not the above approach would be applicable for a particular child at all, would of course depend on the special circumstances of the child with regard to age, type of lesion, cause of lesion, and so forth. In general, the main point to be established here is that consideration of the unilaterally postnatally brain-damaged child offers, in terms of hemisphere disconnection, alternative ways of thinking about possible new therapeutic techniques, and conceptually offers a different way to approach these problems of abnormal brain neurology.

New Directions

The many studies considered in this book, in addition to numerous others, clearly spell out most of the boundary conditions of the split-brain preparation. In some sense there is, therefore, a certain urgency to consider new directions that split-brain research will take. The following discussion concerns several approaches now being explored. In brief, the research is broken down into two main areas. One approach is to study both the experimental animal and man with the callosum intact. The other is to continue to use the split-brain as a research tool; that is, not to study the problem itself, but to use it as a handy technique with which to examine other questions outstanding in neuropsychology.

In the former category, we are currently investigating callosal information mechanisms in the monkey in the following way. In a previous observation (Gazzaniga, 1966c) it was noted that split-brain monkeys with a massive lesion in one hemisphere involving the frontal, parietal, and temporal lobes behaved as though they were functionally blind. Similar observations have been made in the cat (Sperry et al., 1960). When vision was limited exclusively to the lesioned hemisphere the animal would stumble about in the exercise cage bumping into objects laid in its path. When dark-adapted, it could not follow or track a point source of light with any reliability. It would not reach for juicy morsels of food when hungry and in general showed little or no visual capacity. When using the other hemisphere, responses were completely normal. The animals were followed for approximately 30 days before being sacrificed (Fig. 38). While this observation is of considerable interest in itself, in that it remains completely mysterious what the role of nonvisual cortex is in visual learning or perception, we are using this finding in the present study only to assist us in understanding information-transmission systems across the callosum. The experiment has three main phases.

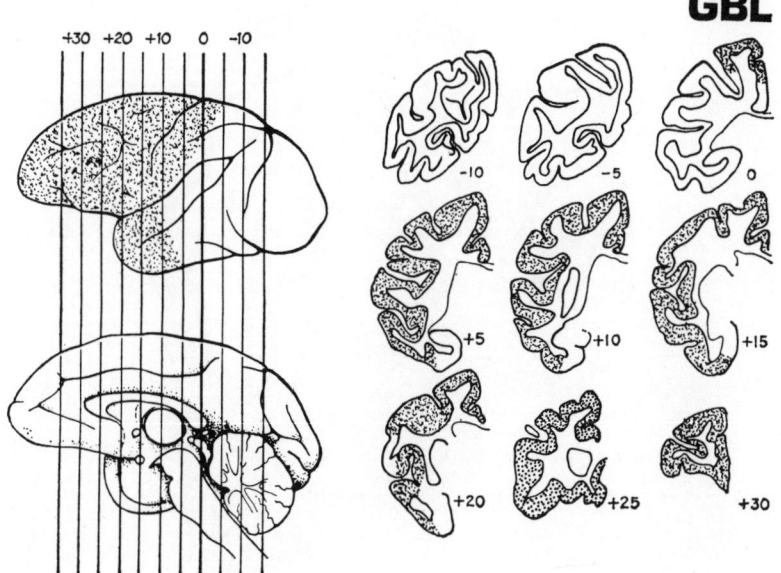

Figure 38. Extent of lesion necessary to produce state of functional blindness in one hemisphere of split-brain monkey.

In the first stage, monkeys undergo midline section of the optic chiasm and anterior commissure. In addition, a small lesion is made in the anterior portion of the callosum. The animals are then trained on a visual discrimination and each eye is tested and shown to be able to perform visual problems. At this point, the animals incur unilateral lesions of the type described above. The entire frontal lobe is removed and considerable damage is inflicted on the postcentral gyrus and infratemporal area. The posterior half of the callosum remains intact, however, and is left largely unaffected by the lesion. After suitable postoperative recovery the visual capacity of each hemisphere is tested. In tests to date, only basic neurologic questions have been examined, with no behavioral data yet available. In brief, when each hemisphere is tested separately it becomes clearly evident that each side can with ease and accuracy guide and control the nonaffected hand. Accurate visual-motor responses are managed by the intact hemisphere as well as by the hemisphere with little visual cortex remaining. The animal shows pupillary responses in both eyes, and each when working alone easily tracks light when dark-adapted.

At this stage the animal undergoes a final surgery, the sectioning

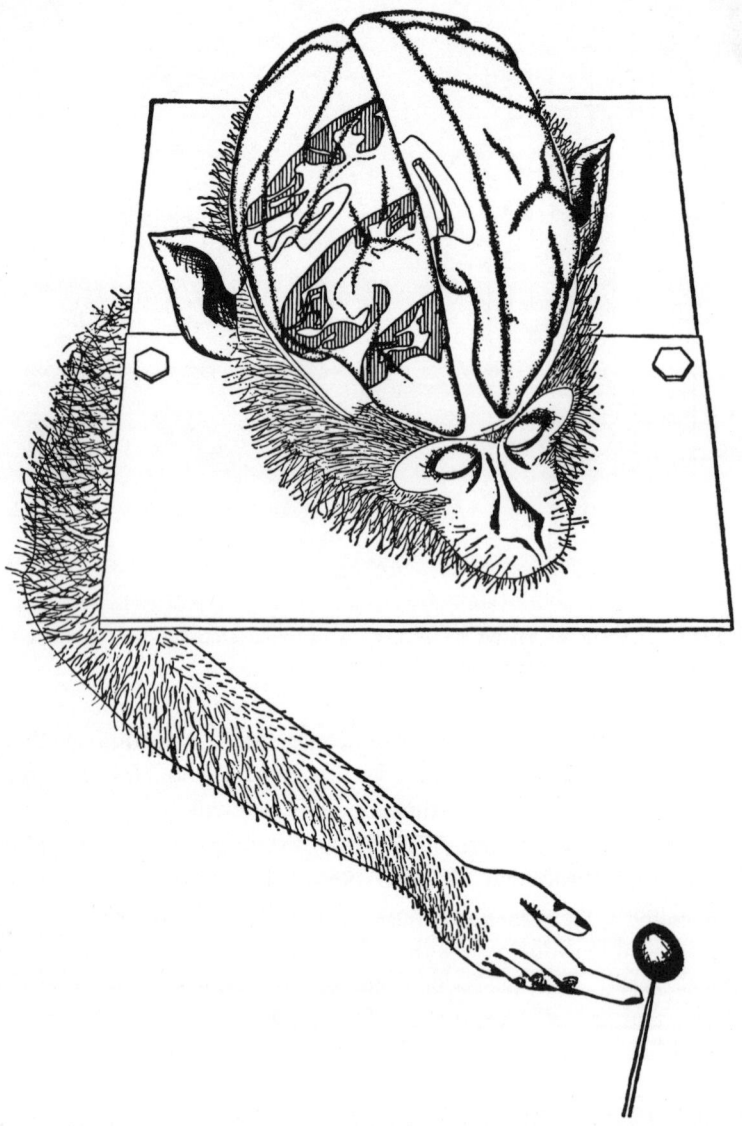

Figure 39. With the left eye occluded, splenium-intact, chiasm-sectioned monkey is able to carry on visually guided behavior with right eye in the presence of a massive lesion as described in Figure 38 and indicated here in cross-section. Following section of the splenium, visual-motor behavior was not possible when using the right eye.

of the posterior half of the callosum (Fig. 39). Again, following an appropriate recovery period, each eye is tested separately.

The lesion-free hemisphere behaves normally, with no deficits observed. Using this half-brain and the contralateral hand, one finds the animal virtually indistinguishable from a normal control.

The lesioned hemisphere, however, behaves quite differently. When it is tested separately, it is now totally unable to direct any kind of visual-motor response. Tantalizing morsels of food positioned immediately in front of the animal fails to elicit any response. When placed in an exercise cage, the animal consistently bumps into obstacles and in general shows no visually guided behavior. When dark-adapted, little or no response is seen to a moving light.

When this rather dramatic behavioral deficit is compared to the level of performance observed when the callosum was present as an input into the lesioned hemisphere, striking differences are of course apparent. These differences, which to date have been defined only grossly, conceivably represent the kinds of information that the splenium is able to transmit. In future tests, the aim will be to further analyze the extent and kind of visual functions present in this preparation with a variety of behavioral tests.

Studies on Normal Man

Today, split-brain research in man, as in experimental animals, is in some instances moving into a new phase. Having established that sectioning the corpus callosum eliminates the interhemispheric spread of high-order information, the task now becomes to study the transmission system itself with the hope that successful analysis of its role in such activities will provide clues on the larger issue of neural encoding of psychologic information. The following represents some initial efforts in this directiton.

When one fixates a point, all visual information falling to the left of fixation is projected to the right hemisphere. Conversely, all information presented to the right of the point is projected to the left hemisphere (Fig. 40). As pointed out in Chapter 6, in a split-brain human this means that a word, say "apple," when flashed in the left visual field, cannot be named or described. The speech mechanism of the left hemisphere is disconnected from the hemisphere that saw the stimulus, namely the right. In normal man, however, the word would easily be

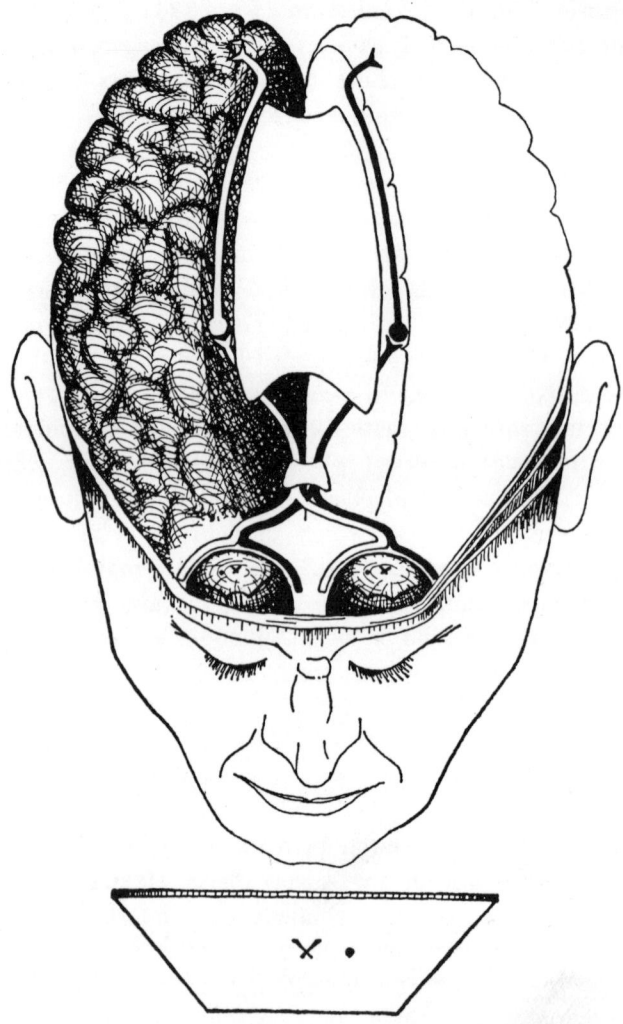

Figure 40. When fixating a point, visual information to the left is normally projected to the right hemisphere. In order for speech comment, the information in some form must be communicated to the left hemisphere via the corpus callosum.

named because the intact corpus callosum would simply relay the information presented to the right hemisphere over to the left, speech, hemisphere. The question becomes, therefore, how and in what form does the corpus callosum transmit such information?

The electrophysiologic studies carried out to date (reviewed in Chapter 5) are not too helpful in coming to an understanding of this problem. In brief, again, the work on the callosum of the cat showed that all the single neurons recorded were activated by stimulation at the midline of the visual field. The recordings that were made in the posterior fifth, or splenium, showed "simple," "complex," and "hypercomplex" types of responses only for areas about the visual midline. This physiology does not help us to understand why we can read and describe things off to one side of the midline or indeed why we are able to verbally describe all information in the left visual half field.

To try to get a better understanding of this general question, we have run a few very simple tests on normal man. In the first test, done in collaboration with Robert Filbey (1969), eight right-handed female students were instructed to fixate a specific point in the visual field when a warning buzzer was presented. Following the flash containing the stimulus, they were instructed to make the appropriate response as quickly as possible and without making an error. A dot or a blank was presented tachistoscopically for 0.1 seconds, being preceded 1.5 seconds by a warning buzzer. The dot was presented either 1 degree to the right or left of fixation. Half of the subjects were instructed to be "dot detectors," verbally responding "yes" to the presence of a dot, and "no" to a blank. The other subjects were instructed to be "blank detectors," responding "yes" to a blank and "no" to a dot presentation. In five days of testing, three banks of twenty trials plus four warm-up trials were run each day. The onset of the test flash started a millisecond timer, which was stopped by a voice-operated relay triggered by the subject's spoken word into a nearby crystal microphone. Error trial times were not recorded nor were the following four trial times, although these latter times were reported to the subject as usual. Following an error and the corresponding four mock trials, testing resumed on the trial following the last recorded correct response. Each day of testing took about 20 minutes per subject. The results of the last two days of testing are tabulated in Table 4.

The data show that when a callosal transmission is necessary for either making the discrimination (as in the case of a blank presentation) or responding appropriately (as in the case of a dot appearing to the left of fixation) reaction times are slower by an average of about 30 msec.

It could be argued that this difference is due to the right cortex simply not being as fast at this kind of task rather than the delay being due to interhemispheric transmission mechanisms. To check this, four right-handed female subjects were used to replicate the previous experi-

TABLE 4. Tests on Eight Female Students (Verbal Report)

Ss	Verbal Response to Dot	Right Dot			Left Dot			Blank		
		Mean of Medians	Mean SD	% Error[a]	Mean of Medians	Mean SD	% Error[a]	Mean of Medians	Mean SD	% Error[a]
MM	Yes	438	37.3	3.2	482	35.8	3.2	458	50.1	0.0
DG	Yes	342	51.8	0.0	388	64.3	0.0	419	64.1	0.0
NS	Yes	284	40.0	0.0	337	52.0	0.0	368	51.6	0.0
SC	Yes	565	76.3	0.0	569	62.7	3.2	592	74.6	1.6
VS	No	359	38.8	0.0	368	31.5	3.2	344	58.8	1.6
CL	No	374	73.7	0.0	422	82.9	6.5	402	49.6	1.6
CF	No	330	58.4	3.2	397	76.7	3.2	364	80.3	0.0
TL	No	388	41.7	0.0	390	55.8	0.0	412	57.0	1.6
Average Over Ss		386	52.2	0.8	419	57.7	2.4	420	60.8	0.8

[a] *Percentage computation does not include mock trials.*

ment. Instead of giving a verbal response, however, they were instructed to give a manual response. This consisted of moving a lever to the right or left, depending on the stimulus. A small displacement of the lever to either side stopped the millisecond timer and turned on a light indicating which response was made. Again, half of the subjects were instructed to be "dot detectors," moving the lever to the right if they detected a dot in the field and to the left following a blank presentation. The remaining subjects were instructed to be "blank detectors," moving the lever to the right following a blank stimulus and to the left for the presence of a dot in the field. The subjects always responded with their right hands.

The results of the last two days of testing are summarized in Table 5. Manual responses to both right and left dots appear to be about equal in the pooled data, while the responses to the blank field are about 40 msec slower on the average.

In studies described in Chapter 4, each hemisphere of a split-brain patient was shown to have good motor control for most responses over either half of the body. Therefore, the experiment using a motor response differs from the one using a verbal response in that in the former both hemispheres have access to the response without using the callosum, while in the latter only the left hemisphere has access to the response. As before, however, callosal transmission is necessary to determine whether or not the entire field was blank. If the results of the first experiment are merely due to peripheral perceptual variables or right cortex inferiority in the task, the results of the second experiment should be identical to those of the first. Clearly, they are not. Using a motor response, reaction times both to a dot to the left and a dot to the right of fixation show little difference, while reaction time to a blank field is, on the average, about 40 msec longer. The data indicate that there exists an intercortical difference in reaction time during a visual pattern discrimination depending on unilateral or bilateral availability of the stimulus and response.

An interesting aspect of the data is the magnitude of differences in reaction time between responses to visual information requiring transmission across the callosum and responses not requiring such transmission. The latency of synaptic transmission is only 0.5 msec, while the differences reported here are in the 30 to 40 msec range. Clearly, the information crossing the callosum does not take the form of one discrete signal or of several simultaneous signals alone. Information

TABLE 5. Tests on Eight Female Students (Manual Response)

Ss	Lever Dis- placement Response to Dot	Right Dot			Left Dot			Blank		
		MEAN OF MEDIANS	MEAN SD	% ERROR[a]	MEAN OF MEDIANS	MEAN SD	% ERROR[a]	MEAN OF MEDIANS	MEAN SD	% ERROR[a]
R	Right	252	57.6	0.0	232	47.8	0.0	284	58.4	0.0
K	Right	374	61.3	3.2	420	37.8	0.0	448	72.9	1.6
SB	Right	322	72.4	0.0	354	72.7	6.5	405	43.4	0.0
JH	Right	364	54.0	3.2	418	71.1	0.0	430	74.5	10.0
L1	Left	218	65.5	3.2	272	59.6	6.5	334	80.6	4.8
L2	Left	394	73.8	0.0	352	61.2	3.2	394	89.0	1.6
JC	Left	412	118.0	35.0	340	56.6	12.0	390	104.0	21.0
CC	Left	348	76.6	12.0	338	68.3	0.0	369	75.0	3.2
Average Over Ss		336	72.4	10.0	341	59.4	3.6	382	74.7	8.4

[a] *Percentage computation does not include mock trials.*

transmission for this type of task seems to require several successive signals over one or more neurons.

It remains for future research to explore the nature of these successive signals and finally to designate the actual routing of information within and between hemispheres during a visual discrimination task like the one reported here. Furthermore, now that a base time has been established for callosal transmission in a very simple visual pattern discrimination task, it remains to be determined whether or not this callosal transmission time increases with the complexity of the discrimination. The answer to that question would give evidence as to the amount of processing each side of the cortex does on the discrimination task, i.e., whether the callosal transmission is some sort of "go, no-go" message or an elaborate read-out of raw visual information.

The Split Brain as a Research Tool

As a last note it is hard to resist mentioning some extremely exploratory findings on some biochemical studies carried out on split-brain pigeons. While the very preliminary results are encouraging, the following is not to be taken as findings yet established in any thorough way. The reason for presenting here the rationale and the experimental data collected to date, is that it would seem that the technique ought to pick up something and that perhaps others might see other real possibilities for experimentation.

Studies on brain function using biochemical techniques have in the main emphasized the role that macromolecules themselves might play in the encoding of memory (Hydén, 1967). The assumption, whether implied or explicit, has been that the mental properties of the brain are represented in biochemical information systems rather than reflecting system properties of an analogue or digital information network.

If one rejects this approach and in its place chooses to view biochemical mechanisms as supportive systems for logical neural networks, then biochemical techniques are used and the data are considered only as they reflect on these system properties. Specifically, the idea involves using radioactive precursors of proteins with the aim of demonstrating differential uptake of the labeled compounds in a trained versus an untrained neural system. A differential uptake in turn would reflect a differential rate of neural firing. The labeled compounds then are viewed as "tracers" of psychologic activity, and with careful analysis particular networks in the brain can perhaps be identified and their relation to particular psychologic activity defined.

A cautionary note, of course, would be that the encoding of information in the neural system might take place without a net increase or decrease through time of firing rate, but rather a rearrangement of the spike discharge pattern. If a neuron fired evenly at a rate of 100 pulses per minute in State A, it could fire at the same overall rate in State B, but the distribution of the pulses might be rearranged in bursts followed by periods of inactivity. If encoding of information is carried out in this fashion, it would be unlikely that biochemical procedures would pick up the changes in neural state.

The specific experimental approach uses the split-brain pigeon, thereby allowing within-subject control, and ruling out confusing influences such as stress, different metabolic states, varying levels of motivation, and the like. Such factors are held constant in each hemisphere while limiting visual learning to one side, for the optic nerves of pigeons are entirely crossed. Differences recorded, therefore, between homologous structures with this preparation might more closely reflect real changes due to learning.

Limitation of visual information to one eye is easily accomplished by affixing goggles to the head. Opaque occluders are then attached to either eye at will. The surgery involves midline section of the tectal and posterior commissures. Subsequent to these manipulations, and after a suitable recovery, the animals are maintained at 80 percent of normal weight and are trained to peck a red key.

After a steady response rate has been realized the animals are ready for the critical test session. Prior to the run, the pigeons are injected with an appropriate amount of H^3-leucine. During the subsequent 45 minutes, the behavior program is changed. Reinforcement occurs only after response to the red stimulus and not to a randomly occurring green stimulus presented on the same key. The time limit is necessary so that differential uptake can be caught. Times longer than 45 minutes would probably find the system so heavily labeled that no distinctions would be possible (Zemp et al., 1966).

The animal is subsequently sacrificed, the brain removed, completeness of surgery checked, followed by separation of the right and left tectum, cerebrum, and brain stem for biochemical analysis. At these first stages of the experimental program equal portions of rather large areas of homologous structures were analyzed for differential uptake.

The foregoing experiment has been run in pilot form in our laboratory, and the preliminary results suggest that the optic tectum does differentially take up 15 percent more H^3-leucine and synthesizes it into cytoplasmic protein, than does the corresponding area in the untrained tectum. This very preliminary study has been encouraging. As continued success of the experimental approach permits, the subdivisions for analyses will become smaller and smaller. Following the appropriate assay procedures, the data from the various diced sections of the brain will be used in a reconstruction allowing for estimations of the brain areas active in a given behavioral task.

References

Akelaitis, A. J. 1941. Studies on corpus callosum; higher visual functions in each homonymous field following complete section of corpus callosum. Arch. Neurol. Psychiat. (Chicago), 45:788.
——— 1943. Studies on corpus callosum; study of language functions (tactile and visual, lexia and graphia) unilaterally following section of corpus callosum. J. Neuropath. Exp. Neurol., 2:226.
——— 1944. Study of gnosis, praxis, and language following section of corpus callosum and anterior commissure. J. Neurosurg., 1:94.
——— A. W. Risteen, R. Y. Herren, and W. P. Van Wagenen. 1942. Studies on corpus callosum; contribution to study of dyspraxia and apraxia of corpus callosum. Arch. Neurol. Psychiat. (Chicago), 47:971.
Basser, L. S. 1962. Hemiplegia of early onset and the faculty of speech with special reference to the effects of hemispherectomy. Brain, 85:427–460.
Berlucchi, G. and G. Rizzolatti. 1968. Binocularly driven neurons in visual cortex of split-chiasm cats. Science, 159:308.

REFERENCES

———— M. S. Gazzaniga and G. Rizzolatti. 1967. Microelectrode analysis of transfer of visual information by the corpus callosum of cat. Arch. Ital. Biol., 105:583–596.

Black, P. and R. E. Myers. 1964. Visual function of the forebrain commissures in the chimpanzee. Science, 146:799.

———— and R. E. Myers. 1965. A neurological investigation of eye-hand control in the chimpanzee. In Ettlinger, E. G., ed., Functions of the Corpus Callosum. London, J. A. Churchill, pp. 47–59.

Blakemore, C. 1969. Psychophysical tests in chiasm-sectioned man. (In preparation.)

———— and D. E. Mitchell. 1969. Depth perception and the corpus callosum. (In preparation.)

Bogen, J. E. 1960. Personal Communication.

———— 1969a. The other side of the brain. I. Dysgraphia and dyscopia following cerebral commissotomy. Bull. Los Angeles Neurol. Soc., 34:73–105.

———— 1969b. The other side of the brain. II. An oppositional mind. Bull. Los Angeles Neurol. Soc., 34:135–161.

———— and B. Campbell. 1962. Recovery of foreleg placing after ipsilateral frontal lobectomy in the hemicerebrectomized cat. Science, 135:309.

———— E. D. Fisher, and P. J. Vogel. 1965. Cerebral Commissurotomy: A second case report. J. Amer. Med. Assoc., 194:1328–1329.

———— and M. S. Gazzaniga. 1965. Cerebral commissurotomy in man: minor hemisphere dominance for certain visuo-spatial functions. J. Neurosurg., 23:394–399.

———— and P. J. Vogel. 1962. Cerebral commissurotomy in man. Preliminary case report. Bull. Los Angeles Neurol. Soc., 27:169.

———— and P. J. Vogel. 1963. Treatment of generalized seizures by cerebral commissurotomy. Surg. Forum, 14:431.

Bremer, F., J. Brihaye, and G. Andre-Galisaux. 1956. 2. Physiologie et pathologie du corps callux. Schweiz. Arch. Neurol. Psychiat., 78:31.

Bridgman, C. S. and K. U. Smith. 1945. Bilateral neural integration in visual perception after section of corpus callosum. J. Comp. Neurol., 83:57.

Butler, C. R. 1968. A memory-record for visual discrimination habits produced in both cerebral hemispheres of monkey when only one hemisphere has received direct visual information. Brain Res., 10:152–167.

Butler, S. R., and U. Norrsell. 1968. Vocalization possibly initiated by the minor hemisphere. Nature (London), 220:793–794.

Choudhury, B. P., D. Whitteridge, and M. E. Wilson. 1965. The function of the callosal connections of the visual cortex. Quart. J. Exp. Physiol., 50:214–219.

Conel, J. L., 1941. The Postnatal Development of the Human Cerebral Cortex Vol. 2, The Cortex of the One-Month Infant. Cambridge, Mass., Harvard University Press, 136 pp.

——— 1959. The Postnatal Development of the Human Cerebral Cortex. Vol. 6, The Cortex of the Twenty-Four-Month Infant. Cambridge, Mass., Harvard University Press.

Day, R. 1969. Dichotic testing of split-brain patients. (In preparation.) ration.)

Doty, R. 1969. Butterflies on the brain. (Paper presented at Federation of American Societies for Experimental Biology meeting, Atlantic City, N. J., April 1969. Not published.)

Downer, J. L. de C. 1959. Changes in visually guided behavior following mid-saggital division of optic chiasm and corpus callosum in monkeys *(Maccaca mulatta)*. Brain, 82:251–259.

——— 1962. Interhemispheric integration in the visual system. *In* Mountcastle, V. B., ed., Interhemispheric Relations and Cerebral Dominance. Baltimore, Johns Hopkins Press, pp. 87–100.

Ebner, F. F., and R. E. Myers. 1962a. Corpus callosum and the interhemispheric transmission of tactual learning. J. Neurophysiol., 25:380.

——— and R. E. Myers. 1966b. Direct and transcallosal induction of touch memories in the monkey. Science, 138:51.

Eccles, J. 1965. The brain and the unity of conscious experience. The 19th Arthur Stanley Edding. Memorial Lecture. Cambridge, England. (University Printing House.)

Ettlinger, G. 1959. Visual discrimination following successive temporal ablations in monkeys. Brain, 82:232–250.

——— 1967. Analysis of cross-modal effects and their relationship to language. *In* Millikan, C. H. and Darley, F. L., eds., Brain Mechanisms Underlying Speech and Language. New York, Grune & Stratton, Inc., pp. 53–60.

——— and H. B. Morton. 1966. Tactile discrimination performance in the monkey; transfer of training between the hands after commissural section. Cortex, 2:30–49.

Evarts, E. V. 1968. Relation of pyramidal tract activity to force exerted during voluntary movement. J. Neurophysiol., 31:14–27.

Falconer, M. A. 1967. Brain mechanisms suggested by neurophysiologic studies. *In* Millikan, C. H. and Darley, F. L., eds. Brain Mechanisms Underlying Speech and Language. New York, Grune & Stratton, Inc., pp. 185–190.

Filbey, R. A. and M. S. Gazzaniga. 1969. Splitting the normal brain with reaction time. (Psychon. Sci. In press.)

REFERENCES

Gardner, W. J., L. J. Karnosh, J. R. McClure, C. Christopher, and A. K. Gardner. 1955. Residual function following hemispherectomy for tumour and for infantile hemiplegia. Brain, 78:487.

Gazzaniga, M. S. 1963. Effects of commissurotomy on a pre-operatively learned visual discrimination. Exp. Neurol., 8:14–19.

——— 1964. Cerebral mechanisms involved in ipsilateral eye-hand use in split brain monkeys. Exp. Neurol., 10:148–155.

——— 1965. Psychological properties of the disconnected hemispheres in man. Science, 150:372.

——— 1966a. Interhemispheric communications of visual learning. Neuropsychologia, 4:261–262.

——— 1966b. Interhemispheric cuing systems remaining after section of neocortical commissures in monkeys. Exp. Neurol., 16:28–35.

——— 1966c. Visuomotor integration in split brain monkeys with other cerebral lesions. Exp. Neurol., 16:289–298.

——— 1966d. Unpublished.

——— 1967a. Dyspraxia following division of the cerebral commissures in man. Arch. Neurol. (Chicago), 16:606–612.

——— 1967b. The split brain in man. Sci. Amer., 217:24–29.

——— 1968a. Intermodal transfer in non-literate hemispheres: Monkey and brain bisected man. (Symposium Paper presented at Eastern Psychological Association meeting, April 1968. Not published.)

——— 1968b. Short term memory and brain bisected man. Psychon. Sci., 161–162.

——— 1969. Cross cuing mechanisms and ipsilateral eye-hand control in split brain monkeys. Exp. Neurol., 23:11–17.

——— J. E. Bogen, and R. W. Sperry. 1962. Some functional effects of sectioning the cerebral commissures in man. Proc. Nat. Acad. Sci. U.S.A., 48:1765–1769.

——— J. E. Bogen, ¹ R. W. Sperry. 1963. Laterality effects in somesthesis follov · · cerebral commissurotomy in man. Neuropsychologia, 1:209–215.

——— J. E. Bogen, and R. W. Sperry. 1965. Observations on visual perception after disconnection of the cerebral hemispheres in man. Brain, 88:221.

——— and R. W. Sperry. 1965. Language in human patients after brain bisection. Fed. Proc., 25:522.

——— and R. W. Sperry. 1966. Simultaneous double performance ability following brain bisection in man. Psychon. Sci., 4:261–262.

——— and R. W. Sperry. 1967. Language after section of the cerebral commissures. Brain, 90:131–148.

———— and E. D. Young. 1967. Effects of commissurotomy on the processing of increasing visual information. Exp. Brain Res., 3:368–371.

Geschwind, N. 1965a. Disconnexion syndromes in animals and man. I. Brain, 88:237.

———— 1965b. Disconnexion syndromes in animals and man. II. Brain, 88:585.

———— and E. Kaplan. 1962. A human cerebral deconnection syndrome. Neurology (Minneap.), 12:675.

Glickstein, M., and R. W. Sperry. 1960. Intermanual somesthetic transfer in split-brain rhesus monkey. J. Comp. Physiol. Psychol., 53:322.

Gordon, H. W. and R. W. Sperry. 1968. Lateralization of olfactory perception in the surgically separated hemispheres of man. Neuropsychologia, 7:111–120.

Hall, M. M., G. C. Hall, and P. Lavoie. 1968. Ideation in patients with unilateral or bilateral midline brain lesions. J. Abnorm. Psychol., 73:526–531.

Hamilton, C. R. 1968. Effects of brain bisection on eye-hand coordination in monkeys wearing prisms. J. Comp. Physiol. Psychol., 64:434–443.

———— and M. S. Gazzaniga. 1964. Lateralization of learning of color and brightness discrimination following brain bisection. Nature, 201:220.

———— S. A. Hillyard, and R. W. Sperry. 1968. Interhemispheric-comparisons of color in split-brain monkeys. Exp. Neurol., 21:486–494.

Hewitt, W. 1962. The development of the corpus callosum. J. Anat., 96:355–358.

Hubel, D. H. and T. N. Wiesel. 1962. Receptive fields, binocular interaction and functional architecture in the cat's visual cortex. J. Physiol. (London), 160:106–154.

———— and T. N. Wiesel. 1967. Cortical and callosal connections concerned with the vertical meridian of visual fields in the cat. J. Neurophysiol., 30:1561–1573.

Humphrey, N. K. and L. Weiskrantz. 1967. Vision in monkeys after removal of the striate cortex. Nature, 215:595–597.

Hydén, Holger. 1967. Biochemical changes accompanying learning. In Quarton, G. C., Melwechut, T., and Schmitt, F. O., eds. The Neurosciences. New York, The Rockefeller University Press, pp. 248–286.

Johnson, J. D. and M. S. Gazzaniga. 1969. Cortical-cortical pathways involved in reinforcement. Nature, 223:71.

Kimura, D. 1967. Functional assymetries of the brain in dichotic listening. Cortex, 3:163–178.
Langworthy, O. R. 1933. Development of behavior patterns and myelinization of the nervous system in the human fetus and infant. Carnegie Institute of Washington Publ. No. 433: Contributions to Embryology No. 139.
Lashley, K. S. 1950. In search of the engram. *In* The Neuropsychology of Lashley, McGraw-Hill Book Company.
Lee-Teng, E. and R. W. Sperry. 1966. Intermanual stereognostic size discrimination in split-brain monkeys. J. Comp. Physiol. Psychol., 62:84–89.
MacKay, D. M. 1966. Brain and conscious experience. *In* Eccles, J. C., ed., Brain and Conscious Experience. Berlin, Springer-Verlag.
MacKay, D. M. 1967. Personal communication.
Majkowski, J. 1967. Electrophysiological studies of learning in split-brain cats. Electroenceph. Clin. Neurophysiol., 23:521–531.
Mark, R. F. and R. W. Sperry. 1968. Bimanual coordination in monkeys. Exp. Neurol., 21:92–104.
Maspes, P. E. 1948. Le syndrome expérimental chez l'homme de la section du splénium du corps calleux alexie visuelle pure hémianopsique. Rev. Neurol. (Paris), 80:100–113.
Meikle, T. H., and J. A. Sechzer. 1960. Interocular transfer of brightness discrimination in split-brain cats. Science, 132:734–735.
——— J. A. Sechzer, and E. Stellar. 1962. Interhemispheric transfer of tactile conditioned responses in corpus callosum sectioned cats. J. Neurophysiol., 25:530–543.
Milner, Brenda. 1962. Literality effects in audition. *In* Mountcastle, V. B., ed., Interhemispheric Relations and Cerebral Dominance. Baltimore, The Johns Hopkins Press.
——— 1968. Alterations of behavior produced by left and right hemisphere lesions. (Paper presented at American Psychological Association meeting, San Francisco. Not published.)
——— L. Taylor, and R. W. Sperry. 1968. Lateralized suppression of dichotically presented digits after commissural section in man. Science, 161:184–185.
Mishkin, M. 1966. Visual mechanisms beyond the striate cortex. *In* Russell, R., ed., Frontiers of Physiological Psychology. New York, Academic Press, Inc., pp. 93–119.
Mitchell, D. E., and G. Westheimer. 1968. (In press.)
Myers, Ronald E. 1955. Interocular transfer of pattern discrimination in cats following section of crossed optic fibers. J. Comp. Physiol. Psychol., 48:470–473.

―――― 1956. Function of corpus callosum in interocular transfer. Brain, 79:358.

―――― 1959. Interhemispheric communication through the corpus callosum: Limitations under conditions of conflict. J. Comp. Physiol. Psychol., 52:6–9.

―――― 1961. Corpus callosum and visual gnosis. *In* Fessard, A., Gerard, R. W., Konorski, J., and Delafresnaye, J. F., eds., Brain Mechanism and Learning. Oxford, Blackwell Scientific Publications, p. 481.

―――― 1962. Transmission of visual information within and between the hemispheres: a behavioral study. *In* Mountcastle, V. B., ed., Interhemispheric Relations and Cerebral Dominance. Baltimore, The Johns Hopkins Press., pp. 51–73.

―――― 1964. Function of area 3 in parietal lobe in the monkey. Fed. Proc., 23:395.

―――― 1965. The neocortical commissures and interhemispheric transmission of information. *In* Ettlinger, E. G. ed., Functions of the Corpus Callosum. London, J. A. Churchill, pp. 1–17.

―――― and C. O. Henson. 1960. Role of corpus callosum in transfer of tactuokinesthetic learning in chimpanzee. Arch. Neurol. (Chicago), 3:404.

―――― N. McCurdy, and R. W. Sperry. 1962. Neural mechanisms in visual guidance of limb movements. Arch. Neurol. (Chicago), 7:195–202.

―――― and R. W. Sperry. 1953. Interocular transfer of a visual form discrimination habit in cats after section of the optic chiasm and corpus callosum. Anat. Rec., 175:351–52.

―――― and R. W. Sperry. 1956. Contralateral mnemonic effects with ipsilateral sensory inflow. Fed. Proc., 15:134.

Noble, J. 1966. Mirror-images and the forebrain commissures of the monkey. Nature (London), 211:1263–1266.

Penfield, W. and L. Roberts. 1959. Speech and Brain-Mechanisms, Princeton, N. J., Princeton University Press.

Posner, M. I. and R. F. Mitchell. 1967. Chronometric analysis of classification. Psychol. Rev. 74:392–409.

Pribram, K. H. 1960. The intrinsic systems and the forebrain. *In* Field, J., Magoun, H. W., and Hall, V. E., eds., Handbook of Physiology: Neurophysiology, II. Washington, American Physiological Society.

Reitz, S. L. 1968. Effects of serial disconnection of striate and temporal cortex on visual discrimination performance in monkeys. J. Comp. Physiol. Psychol., 68:139–146.

Rose, J. E., and V. B. Mountcastle. 1960. Touch and kinesthesis. *In* Field, J., Magoun, H. W., and Hall, V. E. eds., Handbook of

Physiology: Neurophysiology, II. Washington, American Physiological Society.
Schachter, Stanley. 1967. Cognitive effects on bodily functioning. *In* Glass, David C., ed., Studies of Obesity and Eating in Neurophysiology and Emotion. New York, The Rockefeller University Press.
Schrier, A. M., and R. W. Sperry. 1959. Visuomotor integration with split-brained cats. Science, 129:1275.
Sechzer, Jeri A. 1964. Successful interocular transfer of pattern discrimination in "split-brain" cats with shock-avoidance motivation. J. Comp. Physiol. Psychol., 58:76–83.
——— 1968. Interhemispheric integration and prolonged learning in split-brain cats. Proc. Int'l. Union Physiological Sciences, 7:395.
Semmes, J., S. Weinstein, L. Ghent, and H. L. Teuber. 1960. Somatosensory Changes after Penetrating Brain Wounds in Man. Cambridge, Mass., Harvard University Press.
Smith, A. 1966. Speech and other functions after left (dominant) hemispherectomy. J. Neurol. Neurosurg. Psychiat., 29:467–471.
Sperry, R. W. 1959. Preservation of high-order function in isolated somatic cortex in callosum-sectioned cat. J. Neurophysiol., 22:78.
——— 1961. Cerebral organization and behavior. Science, 133:1749.
——— 1964a. Problems outstanding in the evolution of brain function. [James Arthur Lecture.] New York, The American Museum of Natural History.
——— 1964b. The great cerebral commissure. Sci. Amer. 210:42.
——— 1966. Hemispheric interaction and the mind-brain problem. *In* Eccles, J. C., ed., Brain and Conscious Experience. Berlin, Springer-Verlag.
——— 1968a. Mental unity following surgical disconnection of the cerebral hemispheres. The Harvey Lecture Series, 62:293–323. New York, Academic Press, Inc.
——— 1968b. Plasticity of Neural Maturation. Devel. Biol. (Suppl.), 2:306–327.
——— and S. M. Green. 1964. Corpus callosum and perceptual integration of visual half fields. Anat. Record, 148:339.
——— J. S. Stamm, and N. Miner. 1956. Relearning tests for interocular transfer following division of optic chiasma and corpus callosum in cats. J. Comp. Physiol. Psychol., 49:529–533.
——— R. E. Myers, and A. M. Schrier. 1960. Perceptual capacity of the isolated visual cortex in the cat. Quart. J. Exp. Psychol., 12:65–72.
Stamm, J. S., and R. W. Sperry. 1957. Function of corpus callosum in contralateral transfer of somesthetic discrimination in cats. J. Comp. Physiol. Psychol., 50:138.

Stone, J. 1966. The naso-temporal division of the cat's retina. J. Comp. Neurol., 126:585–600.

Teitelbaum, H., S. K. Sharpless, and R. Byck. 1968. Role of somatosensory cortex in interhemispheric transfer of tactile habits. J. Comp. Physiol. Psychol., 66:623–632.

Trescher, J. H. and F. R. Ford. 1937. Colloid cyst of third ventricle; report of case; operative removal with section of posterior half of corpus callosum. Arch. Neurol. Psychiat., 37:959.

Trevarthen, C. B. 1961. Studies on visual learning in split-brain monkeys. Doctoral dissertation, California Institute of Technology.

——— 1962. Double visual learning in split-brain monkeys. Science, 136:258.

——— 1963. Processus visuels intérhemisphériques localisés dan le tronc cérébral. C. R. Soc. Biol. (Paris), 157:2019–2022.

——— 1968. Two mechanisms of vision in primates. Psychol. Forsch., 31:299–337.

——— 1969. Cerebral midline relations reflected in split-brain studies of the higher integrative functions. (Symposium paper presented at the XIX Int'l. Congress of Psychology, London. Not published.)

Voneida, T. J. 1967. The effect of pyramidal lesions on the performance of a conditioned avoidance response in cats. Exp. Neurol., 19:483–493.

——— and R. W. Sperry. 1961. Central nervous pathways involved in conditioning. Anat. Rec., 139:283.

Westheimer, G., and L. Tanzman. 1956. Qualitative depths localization with diplopic images. J. Opt. Soc. Amer., 46:116–117.

White, R. J., L. H. Schreiner, R. A. Hughes, C. S. MacCarty, and J. H. Gridlay. 1959. Physiological consequences of total hemispherectomy in the monkey. Operative method and functional recovery. Neurology (Minneap.), 6:149.

Whitteridge, D. 1965. Area 18 and the vertical meridian of the visual field. In Ettlinger, E. G., ed., Functions of the Corpus Callosum. London, J. A. Churchill, pp. 115–120.

Yamaguchi, Shun-Ichi, and Ronald E. Myers. 1969. Early versus late forebrain commissure section and interocular transfers of visual learning. (Paper presented at Eastern Psychological Association meeting, Philadelphia, April 1969. Not published.)

Zangwill, O. 1964. The brain and disorders of communication. The current status of cerebral dominance. Res. Publ. Ass. Nerv. Ment. Dis., 42:103.

Zemp, J. W., J. E. Wilson, K. Schlesinger, W. O. Boggan, and E. Glassman. 1966. Brain function and macromolecules, I incorporation of evidence into RNA of mouse brain during short-term experience. Proc. Nat. Acad. Sci. U.S.A., 10:1423–1431.

Index

Agnosia, 74
Agraphia, 74
Akinesis, 77
Anterior commissure. *See* Commissure, anterior.
Apraxia, 39, 74
Auditory comprehension. *See* Language, comprehension.
Auditory integration, 89
Auditory localization, 89
Auditory testing, 89

Bimanual discrimination task, 96
Bimanual responding in localization of touch, 84
Biochemical studies in pigeon, 157
Biochemistry of memory, 157
Brain, as two equal halves. *See* double-brain phenomenon.
Brain-bisected humans
 case histories, 75–81

Brain-bisected humans (*cont.*)
 neurologic effects in, 74, 81
 psychologic effects in, 74
Brain damage
 extracallosal, 88
 rehabilitation of children, 146
 unilateral, 142
 wounds in man, 81
Brightness discrimination, 96. *See also* Double-field stimulation.

Calculation, 124
Callosum. *See* Corpus callosum.
Cerebral dominance. *See* Dominance.
Chiasm. *See* Optic chiasm.
Commissure, anterior, 3, 4
 in cat, 2
 in man, 75
 in monkey, 2, 145, 149
 sectioning of, 77, 78, 92
Commissure, hippocampal, 3

Commissure, posterior, 158
Commissure, tectal, 158
Commissures
  interhemispheric transfer, 3–4
  partial section of. See Partial commissurotomy; Splenium.
  pure lesions in, 99
Conscious experience, 143
Contralateral projection
  of audition, 89
  of somesthesis, 87
Convergent eye movement system, 93, 94
Corpus callosum
  agenesis of, 135, 145–146
  in cross-integration, 82
  development of, 131
  in hemisphere disconnection, 146
  as information transmission system, 1, 3, 4, 148, 151–152
  lesions in 65, 74, 140
  neurophysiology of, 67
  in normal man, 151
  partial section of. See Partial commissurotomy.
  role in speech, 152
  section in cat, 153
  section in monkey, 2
  section in man, 74, 77–78, 92, 142, 151
  in stereopsis, 94
  transmission time. See Information transmission.
Cross-cuing strategies, 88, 146
  in position sense, 85
  in somesthesis, 28, 88, 145
  in vision, 92, 94
  target information carry-over, 47
Cross-integration. See also Cross-cuing strategies; Interhemispheric matching.
  in chimpanzees, 74
  in monkeys, 74
  in somesthesis, 82
Cross-localization
  in epileptic, 80
  in somesthesis, 78, 80, 88
  of pain, 85
  parts of body, 88
  postoperatively, 84
Crossed auditory pathways. See Contralateral projection, of audition.
Cutaneous stimulation. See Somesthesis.

Derepression of prewired circuits, 145, 146

Dominance
  for speech, 147
  theory of, 128
  for visual-motor activity, 147
Double-brain phenomenon, 2, 4, 147
Double-field stimulation, 92, 96

"Echo time"
  right hemisphere function, 142
  temporal-order recall test, 90, 142
Electrophysiologic studies, 152–153
Emotion
  in man, 105
  in monkey, 108
Epileptic seizures, 3, 75
Eye-position, 56

Fixation, 92–96. See also Visual field.
  in stereopsis, 93–94
Fornix, 3, 78
Frontal lobe, 148–149
Functional blindness, 148–149
"Fused" words in auditory testing, 89

Grand mal convulsions, 76

Hemisphere disconnection, 146
Hemispherectomy
  in cat, 81
  infantile hemiplegia, 81
  in monkey, 81
Hippocampal commissure. See Commissure, hippocampal.
H^3-leucine, 158

Infantile hemiplegia, 81
Information transfer, 94
Information transmission
  in corpus callosum, 153, 156–157
  neural encoding of, 151
Infratemporal lobe, 30
  lesions of, 149
  in visual learning, 145
Intellectual faculties
  in brain-bisected man, 109
  in brain-bisected monkey, 112
Interhemispheric eye-hand combinations
  in cat, 35
  in chimpanzees, 37
  in man, 39
  in monkey, 35

INDEX

Interhemispheric matching
 in man, 101
 in monkey, 102
Interhemispheric transfer of learning
 shock avoidance, 66
 tactual, 88
Interhemispheric transfer of visual information, 92, 145
Interhemispheric transmission, 153
Intermanual tasks. See Localization of light touch; Temperature discrimination.
Intermanual tranfer
 in stylus maze problems, 87
 in tactile discrimination, 88
Intermodal association
 in man, 25, 95
 in monkey, 22
Intermodal transfer, 86, 95
Intrahemispheric communication, 146
Intrahemispheric eye-hand combinations, 34
Ipsilateral cuing mechanism. See Cross-cuing strategy.
Ipsilateral projection of sensation, 82, 87, 145

Language comprehension
 of commands, 89
 in left hemisphere, 119
 of parts of speech, 119–120
 in right hemisphere, 119
 of spoken word, 121
 through stereognosis, 122
Language expression
 in left hemisphere, 116
 in right hemisphere, 117
Lateralization. See also Contralateral projection; Ipsilateral projection of sensation.
 of language, 116
 of position sense, 85
 of visual function, 97
Learning
 biochemistry of, 157
 electrophysiology of, 157
Learning curves, 2
Localization of light touch, 82. See also Cross-localization.
 bimanual responding, 84
 different parts of body, 83
 verbal responding, 83

Macular sparing, 92
Massa intermedia, 3, 78

Memory. See also Short-term memory; Temporal-order recall test.
 as biochemical information system, 157
 impairment of, 90
Motor system
 brain "set" by vision, 92
 coordination, 79–80
 ipsilateral fibers, 46, 86
 with pure commissural lesions, 99
 right hemisphere control, 99

Necker cube, 97
Neurosurgical chair, 5

Ocular-motor system, 94
Optic chiasm
 sectioned in man, 93
 sectioned in monkey, 2, 145, 149–150
Optic tectum, 159

Pain sensibility, 85
Parietal lesion, 148
Partial commissurotomy. See also Splenium.
 by agenesis, 146
 by surgery, 63, 145, 149
Pattern recognition, 94, 155
Philosophy, 3–4, 147–148
Position sense, 85
Postcentral gyrus lesion, 149
Pupillary responses, 149

Reaction time, 97, 153, 155
Rehabilitation of brain-damaged children, 146–148
Retinal disparity, 93. See also Convergent eye movement system; Stereopsis.
Right hemisphere function, 142. See also "Echo time."

Sensory-motor function
 control mechanism, 33
 performance, 146
Sensory-sensory integration, 19
Short-term memory
 capacity, 113
 deficit, 142
Spelling, 123

Somatic projection
  contralateral, 3, 81
  electrophysiologic evidence, 82
  ipsilateral, 81, 87
Somatosensory function, 75, 87
Somatosensory testing
  neurologic findings, 81
  psychologic findings, 86, 145
Speech mechanism, 151. *See also* Language, expression.
Splenium, 153. *See also* Electrophysiologic studies; Partial commissurotomy.
  information transmission, 151
  interhemispheric transfer, 4
  in visual-motor behavior, 150
Split-brain surgery
  in cat, 12
  in man, 3, 75
  in monkey, 9
  in pigeon, 13
Stereognostic information, 3
Stereopsis, 93
Strategy. *See* Cross-cuing mechanism.
Somesthesis, 76, 81–82
  laterality, 82
  cortical motor control, 87
  testing of epileptics, 78
Subcallosal connections
  elimination of, 44
  interhemispheric transfer, 92, 145–146
Surgery. *See* Split-brain surgery.
Surgical instruments, 7

Tactual discrimination
  interhemispheric transfer, 146

Tactual discrimination (*cont.*)
  intermodal transfer, 86
  learning in cat, 19
  learning in man, 3, 21, 88
  learning in monkey, 21
  memory problems, 86
  stereognostic information, 3
Temperature discrimination, 84–85
Temporal lobe lesion, 148
Temporal-order recall test, 90, 142
Transfer test, 3

Vascular lesions, 74
Verbal localization, 84, 87, 88
Verbal recognition, 95
Visual cortex, 143, 149
Visual discrimination transfer task
  in cat, 2
  double-brain phenomenon, 2
  information transmission, 153, 157
  manual response, 96, 155
  in monkey, 2, 144, 149
  retrieval test, 94
  verbal response, 153
Visual field
  macular sparing, 92
  projection of, 90–91, 151–152
Visual-motor learning, 96, 147, 149, 155
Visual-spatial task, 97
Visual-tactile tests, 95
Visual testing, 76, 90, 94, 148, 151
Visual-visual retrieval tests, 94

Writing, 99, 118